INEQUALITIES AND AFRICAN-AMERICAN HEALTH

How racial disparities create sickness

Shirley A. Hill

First published in Great Britain in 2016 by

Policy Press
University of Bristol
1-9 Old Park Hill
Bristol BS2 8BB
UK
t: +44 (0)117 954 5940
e: pp-info@bristol.ac.uk
www.policypress.co.uk

North American office:
Policy Press
c/o The University of Chicago Press
1427 East 60th Street
Chicago, IL 60637, USA
t: +1 773 702 7700
f: +1 773-702-9756
e:sales@press.uchicago.edu
www.press.uchicago.edu

© Policy Press 2016

British Library Cataloguing in Publication Data
A catalogue record for this book is available from the British Library.

Library of Congress Cataloging-in-Publication Data
A catalog record for this book has been requested.

ISBN 978-1-4473-2282-5 paperback
ISBN 978-1-4473-2281-8 hardcover
ISBN 978-1-4473-2285-6 ePub
ISBN 978-1-4473-2286-3 Mobi
ISBN 978-1-4473-2283-2 ePdf

Cover design by Soapbox Design
Front cover: image kindly supplied by Soapbox Design, London
Printed and bound in the United States of America

Contents

Preface

This book explores how race and racism have an adverse effect on the health of African Americans. A black–white disparity in health and life span has existed in the US for as long as health records have been kept. Middle-class African Americans often fare better than their low-income counterparts, but social class advantage does not eliminate the black health deficit. The health profile of African Americans has its origins in the physical and mental abuse of black people during slavery, and it was perpetuated by another century of racial segregation, violence, and limited opportunity. Social protest and activism during the civil rights era of the 1960s finally brought an end to legalized racial segregation, including the segregated health care system, but did not lead to racial equity in health outcomes. I argue that these persistent racial disparities in sickness and longevity are largely the result of a pervasively racialized social system in which black people continue to be victimized by demeaning racial stereotypes, discrimination, policies that directly undermine their health, and institutionalized racism. Only in recent decades have social scientists begun to explore the connection between health and race, specifically, why African Americans experience poorer health outcomes than Whites. Social and economic factors explain much of the racial disparity in health: for example, Blacks are less likely to embrace healthy behaviors, and are three times more likely than Whites to live in poverty and twice as likely to be jobless. Growing up in economically disadvantaged families and neighborhoods predicts poorer health in adulthood even for those who have achieved socioeconomic mobility. Racial disparities in income, wealth, and status between black and white people in the middle class also help explain why social class does not eliminate racial differences in health outcomes. Researchers have also found that African Americans as a group simply do not get the same quality of health care as Whites, regardless of social class background.

Explanations of racial disparities in health have often emphasized racial differences in health behaviors, health literacy, access to adequate medical care, and interactions between black patients and health care professionals—all-important indicators of how race matters in health outcomes. In this book, however, I argue that these studies fall short of capturing the broader impact on health of living in a racialized social system which maintains existing power relations by perpetuating stereotypes and second-class citizenship for African Americans. This racialized system has an adverse effect on the health of Blacks as they move through multiple settings over their lifecourse, such as schools and the workplace.

Racism and racial stereotypes have a destructive impact on the intimate and marital relationships of African Americans and challenges their ability to create stable families and provide for their children. Social relationships are now widely recognized as important factors in health and wellbeing, but racist policies and racialized gender stereotypes that date back to slavery still undermine the relationships of African Americans. Blacks have fought valiantly for equality, yet many remain at the economic margins of society and are often unable to conform to mainstream gender and family conventions. Many of the hopes of the civil rights era seemed to vanish with the evolution of the post-industrial economy of the 1970s, which took a great toll on African-American marriages and families. This economic downturn resulted in a crisis that was addressed primarily through punitive drug laws and welfare reform policies, resulting in mass incarceration and a host of health issues that affect African Americans across social class and generational boundaries.

This book aims to provide a comprehensive analysis of the factors that perpetuate the black-white disparity in health, health outcomes, and longevity. Part One places the racialized social system in historical context and examines how it affected African-American health from slavery through the 1960s. Part Two focuses on how current social forces create inequities in health, and includes a discussion of the health behaviors of African Americans, the broader social and cultural context that influences those behaviors, and the impact of health policies. Part Three examines the health of African Americans within the context of the post-industrial economy, specifically focusing on the consequences for families of the drug epidemic of the 1970s and 1980s and mass incarceration.

Introduction

At age 59, Russell Stone, an African-American male, believes his health is rapidly failing him and blames most of it on getting old. He has good health insurance—both through his employer and as a military veteran—but is dealing with "blood issues and prostate issues" that are possibly related to having high blood pressure and cholesterol, although his doctors are unable to come up with a specific diagnosis or treatment plan. Russell is worried and frustrated; he knows it is common for people to die before they "make it through their 50s." His brother died at an early age of prostate cancer, and he is concerned that it could happen to him:

> They [the doctors] do tests and things, but they don't know. I was told by one doctor that having to go to the restroom 3-4 times a night was normal, but another [doctor] said it wasn't. I recently blacked out, and I don't know why.... I told my doctor, who said it was kind of normal for men to go through things like that. But I'm getting old, turning 60. A lot of people I know didn't make it through their 50s. My one brother passed away from an enlarged prostate, prostate cancer. I don't know what's going on.

Examined from a medical perspective, Russell's health complaints and inability to have them effectively addressed by doctors is not that unusual. Doctors are often confronted with patients who have an array of ambiguous and fleeting symptoms that defy easy diagnosis, especially when the patient has co-morbidities. Even major chronic illnesses, like multiple sclerosis, can be difficult to diagnose in their early stages. Moreover, most health care professionals these days understand that social factors, such as personal and family relationships, economic hardships, and stressful living conditions can have an adverse effect on the health of their patients, but what can they do about that? Physicians are trained to deal with medical events rather than the life situations that foster them; they simply lack the time, resources, and often interest to deal with the social context of illness.

In recent years the appeal of the biomedical model of illness, the foundation of scientific medicine and the modern health care system, has diminished. Although millions of dollars are still invested in the search for "magic bullets" that will cure specific diseases, the disease burden and our understanding of what causes sickness have changed. Chronic illnesses are, and for decades have been, the leading causes of sickness, disability, and death in the US and other advanced nations, despite the extensive media attention and alarm over occasional surges in infectious diseases. While the latter may be more amenable to effective medical interventions, biomedical science can often neither explain the etiology of a chronic illness nor offer a cure. Sicknesses are caused by an interaction between genetic, environmental, and social conditions, and many defy easy remedies. Patients are increasingly urged to manage their own sicknesses through health and lifestyle changes, but this advice does little to address the underlying and often longstanding social conditions that cause and perpetuate illness.

The social causation of sickness has now become the dominant theory in medical sociology (House, 2001; Phelan et al, 2010), and is especially applicable in advanced Western nations where improved sanitation, an overall higher standard of living, medical technologies, and expanded access to health care have eliminated neither sickness nor persistent racial and social class disparities in health. Numerous studies have shown that low-income and poor people experience higher rates of sickness and early death, and that they engage in riskier health behaviors, such as smoking. The focus on health behaviors, however, often masks the social conditions and inequalities that contribute to those behaviors, such as illness-producing living and working conditions and stressful social relationships. Although he does not situate his health complaints in a social context, Russell's biography reveals a lifetime of adverse life experiences that began in childhood and have extended into his adult years.

Early childhood travails and family instability have an adverse impact on health that lasts through the life course, and Russell has had such experiences. His mother had eight children by three different men; he described her as a "rolling stone" who spent very little time raising any of her children. The composition of the household he grew up in shifted constantly, as his siblings and relatives moved in and out. When he was 10, his biological father deserted the family; a few years later his father died of alcoholism.

At age 17 Russell witnessed the death of his closest friend, who was shot during a minor altercation. He called it a defining moment in his life, explaining that he tried hard to live his life in a way to make his friend proud. Russell joined the military but was discharged early due to a knee injury. Back home, he managed to get into an apprenticeship program in the mid-1970s—an era when the trade unions were accepting more racial minorities—and began to train as a sheet metal worker. Three of the 40 men accepted into the apprenticeship program were African American, and two of the three managed to complete the training. Russell was one of them, and he achieved some financial mobility, married, and bought a home. But the job took a toll on him; he was continually being laid off for long periods of time and subjected to discrimination when he did have work. As Russell explained:

> Discrimination is stressful, not being treated fairly. That can be very stressful. That happened a lot … it's a good old boys club, and we [black men] were the lowest on the totem pole. It was designed to keep us out—we weren't meant to make that kind of money. My journey of being an apprentice wasn't fair. You see them teach others [Whites] how to read blueprints, while they ask you to sweep the floor. You're always trying to get a Caucasian to see the potential in you. So it was a journey like that. No matter what I did, it wasn't right. We did what we were told, then the big boss would come through and say it wasn't right … [that] we should have known better. The union couldn't do anything for me.

Thus, added to a lifelong set of social conditions that would affect the health of practically anyone, Russell believes he was the victim of overt racial discrimination. He finally quit the job and the union, a few years short of being able to draw retirement benefits:

> I needed a year or two to work before I could retire with benefits, but I couldn't wait. For a whole seven long years, I didn't work at all—laid off. I was always laid off around Christmas—didn't have the money to buy the kids stuff.

Russell now holds a janitorial position at a hospital. The work is steady and the pay and benefits are okay, but the job does not represent the upward mobility he had sought to achieve. Downward mobility has an adverse effect on health, while people who experience upward mobility in their work careers live longer, healthier lives (Pavalko and Caputo, 2013). There have also been disappointments in his family life.

Although Russell never wanted to create the type of family he grew up in, he has had three failed marriages and fathered two sons. He is engaged to be married again and, asked who he relies on for social support, named his fiancé. His major sources of stress now are "finances, and other people's issues." Although he works full-time and his fiancé works part-time, they are still trying to put together the money they need to get married. Family relationships remain a major source of stress for Russell: most of his siblings live nearby, and Russell reaps the benefits and social stress of his extended family. He laments rarely getting to see any of his five grandchildren because his sons are estranged from the children's mothers, and is frustrated over having to support his 57-year-old brother who "still hasn't figured out life yet." In this context, it is perhaps not surprising that Russell struggles with several health challenges.

Purpose of the book

This book explores how the health of African Americans is influenced by numerous social settings and policies that reinforce racial inequality. The major argument is that African Americans live in a pervasively racialized society where blackness signifies racial inferiority and leads to policies, attitudes, and stereotypes that adversely affect every aspect of black life, fostering sickness and early death. By racialized society, I refer to a nation where race is deeply embedded in the national consciousness, where black lives are routinely disrespected and devalued, and where black people are perpetually in marginal or subordinate positions. This creates a chronically stressful environment for African Americans across social class boundaries and diminishes their health and life chances.

The majority of African Americans can recount at least one incident of racial discrimination, and research shows that such incidents have an adverse effect on their emotional and physical health. Nevertheless, these isolated incidents fall short of capturing the myriad ways in which racism and racial stereotypes play out in multiple social settings over the course of a lifetime (for example, schools, public spaces, the medical system, the criminal justice system), and are institutionalized in practices and policies. Research on how race and racism affect health has often focused on health- and medical-related factors, such as access to medical care, health behaviors, and provider-patient interactions.

This research has yielded many valuable findings and documented the fact that African Americans simply do not receive the same quality of medical care as White Americans. However, narrowly linking specific health outcomes (for example, depression) with specific aspects of medical care (for example, perceptions of racism) fails to capture the broader racialized social settings. Medical sociologists these days argue that social conditions affect health more than medical care (Phelan et al, 2010; Marmot, 2015), and have linked sicknesses to chronic stress, especially stress that is not easily mediated by coping resources (Pearlin, 1989).

The objective of this book is to provide a comprehensive analysis of how racial disadvantage affects the health of African Americans. Existing research has begun to identify the individual and structural factors that contribute to the health deficit experienced by African Americans. I build on that research and situate it within the broader context of the corrosive effect of a racialized social system on the health of black people. Central to my analysis is examining race in historic and contemporary context and delineating the ways in which racism and stereotypes contribute to poor health among African Americans. I also pay attention to how inequalities based on social class and gender affect health, but prioritize the analysis of racial inequality because it rarely receives adequate attention. Although research is beginning to look at the independent impact of racial inequality on health, it is still common to conflate race, class, and culture, thus evading the topic of racial oppression and leaving discussions of race and health relegated to small sections of textbooks that provide health profiles of "people of color." Thus, I hope to elevate race to a more prominent place in the study of health inequalities.

This book integrates and expands on existing literature to provide a broad analysis of African-American health. I draw on 37 interviews with a class-diverse group of African-American women and men that I conducted explicitly for the purpose of this book to explore health attitudes and experiences. More marginally I draw on interview data I have collected over the years on black families and health. This book examines the impact of the medical system and medical encounters on health, but gives equal consideration to how race and racism undermine intimate relationships and families that often foster good health and healthy environments for rearing black children.

Overview of the chapters

This book offers a broad integrative analysis of the health of African Americans within the context of a racialized social system that affects every aspect of black life and has significant health implications. It is divided into three parts and seven chapters. Part One, which contains the first two chapters, is devoted to providing a historical foundation for the analysis. In Chapter One I describe the origin of the concept of race in Western society and how it was, for centuries, understood as a biological category and used to justify the subordination, oppression, and economic exploitation of African Americans. Slavery and racial segregation were the law of the land for nearly 350 years, establishing the foundation for the racialized social setting of contemporary society. Only in the mid-20th century, with legal segregation still in place, did scholars begin to contend that race was a socially constructed category rather than a biological fact. Amid social protests and demands for racial justice, equal opportunity laws were passed, and many African Americans experienced socioeconomic mobility. However, as I highlight in this chapter, this did not end the racialized social system that continues to disadvantage black people. I discuss the growing intraracial diversity among black people based on social class mobility, immigration, and interracial unions, and the health implications of that diversity. Chapter One concludes with an elaboration of how the racialized social system continues to have an adverse effect on the lives of African Americans.

The health deficit experienced by African Americans cannot be solely explained by their current life situations, as it is rooted in slavery, emancipation, and racial segregation, all of which fostered racial disparities in health. Although the historic health experiences of African Americans have received some recent attention, they are notably absent from research that describes health patterns or the evolution of the health care system. Chapter Two helps write the experiences of African Americans into the study of health, medicine, and the formation of the modern health care system. I draw on historical data to describe the dire living and working conditions endured by enslaved Africans and place it within the broader context of health in colonial America, but also focus on how racism, slavery, and the harsh and injurious punishment doled out to control slaves affected their health (Baptist, 2014).

Emancipation presented yet another health crisis for black people, as it reduced even the meager care slaves might have had when they were defined as the "property" of their owners (Downs 2012). Modern medicine was in its nascent stages when slavery was abolished, but gave scientific merit to theories of racial inferiority and, after slavery ended, racial degeneracy among African Americans. Scientific medicine used the bodies of enslaved black people and other poor folk for medical experiments and the practice of surgery, leaving many African Americans afraid of white physicians for years to come. This chapter examines the struggle for health care equality, the eventual emergence of an integrated health care system, and greater opportunity for African Americans to pursue careers in medicine.

Part Two of the book focuses on health behaviors, health settings, and black people's interactions with the medical system. In the current post-medical era, where the leading causes of sickness and death are from chronic illnesses that are often more preventable than curable, the study of health behaviors has become a major topic among medical sociologists. Chapter Three draws on interview data to examine how African Americans define health and engage in health behaviors to protect their health. This "ethos of healthicization," however, promotes the ideal of individual responsibility for one's health, and runs the risk of blaming people for their sickness. This chapter draws on two models of health lifestyles—the health belief model and the theory of health lifestyles—to explain how people make decisions about taking care of their health and how those decisions are shaped by the broader social context, specifically, religious institutions and neighborhoods.

Chapter Four shifts the focus to illness behaviors—for example, how people respond to symptoms of sickness—and health care policies. This chapter draws on my research on sickle-cell disease, a chronic illness that in the US primarily affects African Americans, to show how race shapes responses to symptoms of illness. The bulk of the chapter, however, explores the factors that impede or facilitate access to quality health care for African Americans. A key factor in the racial disparity in medical care is that black people are less likely to have private insurance than white people and more likely to access care in the public sector of the health care system. But race also shapes the assumptions physicians make about their patients and the treatment options offered.

Racial disparities in health are related to inequalities in the medical system, but more broadly in other social institutions, and none is more important than the family. Part Three of the book looks at how race and racialized policies affect black families, intimate relationships, and children. Families are vital to the health and welfare of their members, but slavery and racial segregation historically undermined the stability and functionality of African-American families. The civil rights era brought new hope to many African Americans, but a decade later the post-industrial economic decline had begun to take a toll of Blacks' opportunities for employment and marriage. This decline affected American families across racial boundaries, but the greatest impact was on those who were already at the economic margins, especially African Americans. High rates of joblessness and idleness among young black men led to an explosion of drug trafficking and crime in urban areas, and draconian policies of welfare reform and incarceration were enacted that disproportionately affected black families. Chapter Five looks at how criminal activities and the policies passed to control them affected African Americans across social class and generational boundaries.

Chapter Six focuses on the health implications of sexuality and intimate relationships between African Americans. Love, social relationships, and social support have a powerful impact on health, but the ability to achieve healthy relationships is undermined by social class and racial inequalities. The longstanding tradition of "love and trouble" between black men and women, based largely on the inability of many to conform to culturally dominant expectations about gender and families, has intensified in an era of economic decline. Marriage has never been as fully institutionalized among African Americans as it has among Whites and, although rates of marriage have now have fallen for all Americans, they have done so more drastically for Blacks. For many, intimate relationships have become more fleeting and often more exploitative, with significant health consequences for men and women.

African-American children are especially affected by the marital and family patterns of their parents, and their health is the topic of Chapter Seven. This chapter examines how parents evaluate the health of their children and the health and sexual socialization they provide for them. The latter is especially important, given the health risks of early pregnancy and the proliferation of sexually transmitted diseases among young African Americans. Most parents love their children and do their best to take care of them, but structural factors matter. Although thousands of children who grow up in low-income single-parents households go on to lead successful lives, a growing body of literature supports the idea that those who grow up in a household with both biological parents fare better. In recent years, government support for the welfare of children has waned, and a significant proportion of children grow up in poverty and low-income households, including more than half of all African-American children. These children are doubly disadvantaged by class and race. Most black parents understand that their children are exposed to denigrating racial stereotypes, and they try to racially socialize their children. These efforts, however, may be countered by living in poor, high-risk neighborhoods that reinforce theories of racial inferiority and attending schools where they are not expected to succeed. These early environments, Neal Halfon has argued, literally "get under a child's skin," and predict health problems throughout life (Halfon, 2012). The Conclusion calls for a greater understanding of how racism damages the health of all Americans and a focus on addressing the social conditions that undermine health.

Part One
Theorizing social inequalities in health

The more than 40 million African Americans who live in the US carry a disproportionate share of the nation's sickness burden. Sociologist David R. Williams, who has written extensively about the black-white health disparity, has repeatedly shown that African Americans not only have higher rates of sickness than Whites, but they also get sick earlier, have more severe diseases, and are more likely to die from their diseases (Williams and Sternthal, 2010; Williams, 2012; Williams and Mohammed, 2013). Black people have higher rates of death than Whites for 13 of the 15 leading causes of death, and they have more nonfatal diseases (Hayward et al, 2000). Heart disease and cancer, the two leading causes of death, strike African Americans at an earlier age and result in more premature deaths. These racial disparities in health start at the moment of birth: black infants are more likely than white infants to be born preterm and underweight, to have more developmental problems, and to die in infancy (Rosenthal and Lobel 2011). The health disadvantages of early childhood persist throughout life, leading to poor health, more functional limitations, and earlier death among African Americans; they also curtail educational attainment and career mobility (Garbarski, 2014; Umberson et al, 2014; Rossin-Slater, 2015).

The earliest systematic data available on race and health date back to the 1800s, and consistently document the black health deficit. Sickness and early death, however, were common during that era, and the fact that African Americans were sicker and died earlier supported theories of their innate, biological inferiority. Sociology emerged during that time as the study of modernity with a focus on how social environmental forces transformed societies, but early theorists expressed little interest in how those forces affected health (Gerhardt, 1989). Many were concerned about the transformations caused by industrialization, such as increases in family and community instability and socially deviant behaviors, but gradually came to understand modernity as evolution toward a more highly developed society. Structural-functionalism became and remained the dominant theoretical paradigm among US sociologists until the late 1950s, focusing on how macro level forces were modernizing societies, institutions, and cultural values. Structural functionalism resonated with the "American Dream" ideology of upward mobility for everyone who worked hard to achieve it, but it also held essentialist notions of race and gender that led to virtually ignoring people of color and women.

Sharply contrasting this perspective was the work of Karl Marx and Friedrich Engels, who offered scathing critiques of how industrial capitalism was undermining the health of the working-classes (Engels, 1892). The mass of industrial workers lived in ever-deepening poverty and misery and suffered from high rates of infectious diseases and premature death due to the inhumane living and working conditions that were forced upon them—for example, high levels of air pollution, inadequate ventilation in factories, and poor sanitation. These theorists argued that industrial Western nations were dominating the global economy because they benefited immensely from slavery and exploiting the labor and resources of people in poor nations. This critique of industrial capitalism never gained much traction in the US, however, although the public health movements of the late 1800s at least tacitly recognized the link between social environmental conditions and health. That focus waned, however, with the discovery of the germ theory of disease and, by the 1950s, the booming post-war economy that created more social class equality (House, 2001).

Medical sociology originated during this era and, like much of the discipline, did not offer a strong critique of structural inequalities in health. Some medical sociologists acknowledged social class-based disparities in health and health behaviors, but their work often focused on white ethnic groups and sought to understand how they responded to symptoms of illness (Zborowski, 1952; Zola, 1966). Their work was insightful, but far from a critique of structural inequalities in health or access to health care. Not until the 1960s did a more critical perspective emerge among medical sociologists, and it primarily challenged the organization and power of the medical system.

Symbolic interactionism has roots as deep as structural functionalism but focuses more on micro-level human interactions and processes. From this perspective human beings have agency in defining and creating reality, and those realities have important consequences for shaping societies and the experiences of individuals. Drawing on this perspective medical sociologists challenged the idea that the biomedical model of illness was based on objectivity and scientific neutrality, arguing instead that medical knowledge and diagnoses were as much a matter of social construction as a biological fact (Gerhardt, 1989). Theorists contended that in its effort to find and eradicate disease, medical science often constructed conditions that did not formerly exist (Freidson, 1970), and they pointed to the growing medicalization of social life and problems (Conrad and Schneider, 1980). Sociologists also became more likely to embrace conflict theory, especially in criticizing the existence of a profit-driven, capitalist medical system that defined health as a commodity to be purchased rather than a right of citizenship.

The women's health care movement emerged in this era of protest and drew on symbolic interactionism and conflict theory to criticize gender inequities in health and the organization of the health care system. Its key premise was that gender is socially constructed in a way that adversely affects women, their health, and their participation in the medical system. Although the higher rates of sickness that women experience may have some basis in biology, they argued that gender norms and stereotypes adversely affected women's health by constraining their full participation in society (Bird and Rieker, 2008). Moreover, medical knowledge about women's health was saturated with sexist and essentialist theories that ignored the link between their life experiences and their health and medicalized female functions such as childbirth (Ehrenreich and English, 1978). The problem also reflected the gender hierarchy in medicine, where physicians were overwhelmingly white men from privileged backgrounds (Zimmerman and Hill, 2000).

The feminist critique of the health care system was pivotal in generating a discussion of the impact of social inequalities on health, but it was evident that the experiences of middle-class white women were different from those of low-income and women of color. The latter experienced issues such as the lack of access to adequate medical care, disrespect from health care professionals, and violations of their reproductive rights. These class and racial inequities had already propelled black female activism, which started in the early decades of the 20th century and promoted individual and social interventions to improve black health (Smith, 1995). In the 1970s, Byllye Avery, an African-American health activist, founded a clinic in Gainsville, Florida devoted to addressing black women's health issues. The National Black Women's Health Project officially started in 1984, with the goal of empowering women with control over their lives and health (Morgen, 2002). Social class and racial differences in health issues pointed to the need for an intersectionality perspective that theorized race, class, sexuality, and gender intersecting inequalities in the production of health inequalities (Collins, 1990). Still, "gender" typically centered only on women and ignored male experiences and perspectives.

Social inequalities in health have now become a major focus in medical sociology, and social conditions as the fundamental cause of sickness and death has become the major theory in the field (Link and Phelan, 1995; Phelan et al, 2010). This theory is especially applicable in advanced societies where improved sanitation and modern health services, and even universal health care, have not eliminated racial and social class disparities in morbidity and mortality. That social conditions are the fundamental cause of sickness had become so irrefutable that a 1995 edition of the *Journal of Health and Social Behavior*, celebrating 40 years of medical sociology, was devoted to the topic. Link and Phelan have argued that medical sociology has devoted too much attention to identifying individual risk factors that affect health, such as smoking, diet, and exercise, but far too little to understanding how social conditions affect health and health behaviors. Moreover, they pointed out that although the link between social conditions and class is apparent, much more research needs to be done to show how social conditions affect gender and racial health inequalities (quoted in Masters et al, 2015).

Research in medical sociology on racial inequalities and health, in fact, remains in its nascent stages, despite the revolutions of the 1960s, changing racial ideologies and the fact that the black–white color line essentially defined racial boundaries. James House pointed out that the first edition of the popular *Handbook of medical sociology* (published in 1963) did not even list the words "poverty," "black," or "Negro" in its index (House, 2001). Not until 2000 did this often-updated and popular textbook include a chapter that explicitly dealt with racial and social class disparities in health. In his examination of the contributions of medical sociology to understanding racial disparities in health, D. R. Williams also found that prior to 1990, major sociological journals had at best only a handful of articles about race and health (Williams and Sternthal 2010). The health experiences of African Americans are also missing from theories and concepts generated by medical sociologists, such as the sick role concept and medicalization. The next two chapters advance the study of race and health by examining how social definitions of race create disadvantage and influence health, thus placing the health deficit of African Americans in historic perspective.

ONE

Race, racism, and
health outcomes

That patterns of health, sickness, and mortality vary on the basis of race is irrefutable, and this has made race a major 'variable' in research in the medical and health sciences. Cross-national data reveal that in every race-conscious nation in the world, racially dominant groups are healthier and live longer than racially subordinate groups (Williams, 2012). But what is race? And through what mechanisms does it affect health? Definitions of race have shifted in recent decades, and it is now seen as more of a socially defined category than a biological fact. That race is a social construct has been widely—although not universally—accepted among scholars, and this has offered new possibilities for rethinking the meaning of skin color and phenotype. However, it has neither erased damaging racial stereotypes about African Americans nor has it eliminated racial discrimination. Although the majority of Americans today endorse racial equality and equal opportunity, black people encounter race-based disadvantages over the course of their lifespans and in multiple settings. In the pervasively racialized social system of the US, whiteness still symbolizes goodness, morality, intelligence, and attractiveness, and blackness is seen as the absence of those attributes.

Research has shown that despite widespread support for racial equality, many white people still hold a spate of racial stereotypes about black people (for example, they are lazy, prone to violence, immoral). They may be less likely to explain their beliefs in terms of biological factors, but equating blackness with inherently flawed social and cultural values is no less damaging. An example of this is found in a quote from a white male asked to explain racial inequality:

I think the majority [of black people] aren't enthused, not motivated, and don't care. The opportunity is there if they want to take advantage. I don't think most Blacks want to work for anything. (quoted in Kwate and Meyer, 2010: 1833)

African Americans are intensely aware of racism and racial stereotypes, and more than 90 percent report that they have experienced racial discrimination (compared to 10 percent of Whites) (Bratter and Gorman, 2011). History reveals a continuous struggle by African Americans to resist oppression and discrimination, yet pervasive racism still fosters psychological and physical violence; it does so even more insidiously when it is institutionalized into social policies that adversely affect the life chances of black people. Racism is a chronic stressor for African Americans, whether it is ignored, challenged, or internalized, and it poses significant barriers to their ability to achieve socioeconomic success or to abide by dominant cultural values. Social class and racial inequalities, in fact, have been pivotal in developing the stress paradigm in medical sociology (House, 2001). Theorists have documented a direct link between social stress and sickness, with stressful life events predicting illnesses as serious as heart disease. They have also pointed out that chronic life strains diminish feelings of self-esteem, self-worth, and the sense of mastery over life, and thus have a detrimental impact on health. Life strains that are deeply entrenched in the social and economic organization of life are often impervious to individual coping efforts. They confront people with "dogged evidence of their failures," according to Pearlin, "and inescapable proof of their inability to alter unwanted circumstances in their lives" (Pearlin et al, 1981: 340).

This chapter begins with a discussion of the origins of race as a biological concept and the emergence of a sociological perspective that defined race as a socially constructed category, but one with immense social and political consequences. Much evidence supports the socially constructed nature of racial categories, including the growing racial diversity of the black population, which has reshaped the relationship between race and health. This growing diversity has further challenged the notion of biological race, but has not eliminated the racialized social system that is rooted in notions of black inferiority. I examine how this racialized social system fosters social class disadvantage and promotes structural violence against African Americans. The persistent relegation of black people to the economic and social margins of society strengthens racist ideologies and, for African Americans, elevates the fears, uncertainties, and racial injustices that create stress and the social conditions that adversely affect health.

Race: historical foundation

Social scientists associate race with physical characteristics (for example, skin color, hair texture) that stem from national origins and biological ancestry and ethnicity with cultural characteristics. The two concepts often, but not always, overlap. The focus in early sociological research was mostly on ethnicity and was driven by the stream of white ethnic immigrants from southeastern Europe who came to the US during the early 20th century. They were racially and culturally distinct from the earlier English settlers in many ways, but especially language and religion, and were expected to undergo a process of assimilation to take on the dominant American culture. Studies of ethnic assimilation were popular in sociology during the early to mid-20th century; however, they were largely inapplicable to African Americans who were involuntary immigrants and expected to "stay in their place" rather than assimilate. Slavery and racial segregation were justified by theories of black racial inferiority, and penalties for transgressing rigid racial codes and boundaries were often severe.

The concept of race has its origins in 15th-century exploration, when European Whites first encountered people of color across the globe—the "cultural other"—and judged them as inferior to themselves. People of color became objects of scientific inquiry and exploitation, with ethnocentric Whites theorizing themselves and their culture as racially superior to others. This paved the way for the racial and economic domination of people of color, which intensified when industrial capitalism expanded and required cheap labor. For Africans, this meant centuries of slavery and virulent forms of racism and oppression that denied their humanity and defined every aspect of their lives. Being defined as black, which meant having any African ancestry, became a master status, despite social and economic distinctions among African Americans, and the black–white color line the most rigidly enforced of all racial distinctions.

Theories of racial inferiority stigmatized and stereotyped African Americans and were almost universally accepted, resulting in laws that severely restricted every aspect of their lives. Most people, including social scientists, accepted race as a biological category and rarely challenged essentialist notions of black racial inferiority. Although Africans came to the US from multiple countries and had a variety of skills, slavery and racial oppression had a homogenizing effect on them as it made blackness their most important characteristic. Even as African Americans moved from slavery to freedom, and from being defined as "property" to second-class citizens in a racially segregated society, they continued to be viewed as intellectually and morally inferior to Whites. Legalized segregation and "Jim Crow" rules reinforced racial inequality and the economic marginalization of African Americans. Racial violence against black people was common, including untold numbers of rapes and beatings, and the documented lynching of more than 6,000 people, few if any of which were effectively addressed by the criminal justice system (Evans and Feagin, 2015).

Social construction of race

The latter half of the 20th century witnessed a seismic shift in our thinking about race and racism, especially as it pertains to African Americans. For a number of reasons—for example, the long history of black resistance to oppression, the racial genocide that occurred during the Second World War in Nazi Germany, and the civil rights movement of the 1960s—scholars began to rethink notions of race, especially the belief that it was based on biological differences. Most scholars came to see race as a social construct, or more of a product of social definitions than biological features. There is little evidence of significant biological or genetic differences between people, but significant support for the social constructionist view of race. From a biological standpoint, there are no "pure races" in the sense of genetically homogeneous populations; in fact, there is little evidence in recorded history that racially pure groups have ever existed.

The social constructionist framework theorizes racial groups as socially created through processes of racialization, or assigning meaning to real, perceived, or ascribed differences between groups, and then making those differences the basis for distributing power and prestige (Burton et al, 2010). People of color in the US have primarily been defined as racial groups—for example, surveys and censuses usually ask people to self-identify based on racial categories. These racial categories do not, however, reflect the level of racial diversity that exists among Americans—for example, people from the Middle East (for example, Arabs, Jews, Iranians), and some Hispanics, are categorized as "White." The racial category "Mexican" was used only in the 1930 federal census, dropped amid protest, and reinstituted in 1970 as Hispanic. Panethnic categories like Asian American also include people from several countries and cultures. And while Jews are usually categorized racially as White, they are in reality an ethnic group that can be composed of various races. Anyone with African ancestry was legally categorized as Negro, Black, or African American.

The social construction of racial categories is seen in shifting definitions of whiteness and even more so in determined efforts to delineate the black–white color line. The rule of hypodescent, also known as the "one drop rule," held that children born of mixed racial unions had to be assigned the race of the racially subordinate parent. The dominant racial hierarchy placed African Americans as subordinate to all other racial groups, and anyone with any known African ancestry was legally categorized as Black. That rule is still commonly applied—for example, Barack Obama, the son of a white mother and black African father, is considered the first black president of the US, despite his mixed racial heritage. Still, African ancestry is not always evident in one's phenotype, and numerous people legally defined as Black have passed for White.

Growing complexity of defining race

The social construction of racial categories has become even more difficult with the growing diversity in the black population. Scholars have noted that since race is socially constructed, the identities and rules associated with it are fluid and subject to change (Burton et al, 2010). This has become more apparent for African Americans in the post-civil rights era because of greater social class diversity, an increase in interracial unions and biracial children, and a growing population of black immigrants from Africa and the Caribbean. Although there has always been some social class diversity among African Americans, being black was once almost synonymous with being poor. In 1940, about 80 percent of black people worked in the three lowest occupational categories (farming, service workers, and laborers), and the majority lived in poverty (Gilbert, 2011). Black people are still overrepresented among the poor—in 2013, nearly 28 percent were poor, compared to 9.8 percent of Whites, but the majority are in the working and middle classes.

Another dimension of intraracial diversity among black people that might affect health is the growth of interracial unions, multiracial people, and the foreign-born black population. A significant number of African Americans have white ancestry, and that number is growing. Interracial marriage has become more common; today, 17 percent of

Blacks marry non-Blacks, a threefold increase since 1980. Interracial people are challenging racial boundaries, as many insist on claiming racial identities that reflect the heritage of both of their parents. The federal census for 2000 was the first to officially acknowledge the multiracial heritage of citizens by allowing the selection of membership in more than one racial group. More than seven million Americans identified as multiracial, leaving nearly 13 percent of all Americans (nearly 40 million people) indicating that they were either black or had black heritage.

Children of black-white unions tend to have a lighter skin tone than other Blacks, and often a phenotype more similar to Whites. Studies of colorism have found that this elevates their status and provides them with special privileges and advantages—among Blacks and in the mainstream White society (Burton et al, 2010). Some of that advantage may be the result of the material and social resources of their parents, often the white parent, since light-skinned minorities are less likely to grow up in poverty or abuse drugs or alcohol and, compared to their darker-skinned counterparts, they earn more money (Burton et al, 2010). Those privileges also appear to have health implications—light-skinned Blacks have lower rates of hypertension than dark-skinned Blacks, which may be related to the fact that the former are less likely to experience racial discrimination (Klonoff and Landrine, 2000).

The foreign-born black population has grown, and black immigrants appear to have a health profile that differs from that of native-born Blacks. Between 1990-2000, there was a 66.9 percent growth in the black immigrant population, raising the number in the US to about three million (Erving, 2011). Some research has found that among people of color, first-generation immigrants have better health than their native born counterparts (Erving, 2011; Williams, 2012). Foreign-born black mothers, for example, are less likely than native-born Blacks to have low weight babies, and have birth outcomes that are more similar to those of white mothers (Deal et al, 2014). In a study comparing native-born Blacks, US-born Caribbeans, and foreign-born Caribbeans, Erving (2011) found that black women across the board had longer life spans than black men, but usually fared worse than men on health outcomes. But native-born black women had the poorest self-assessed health and more functional limitations and serious chronic illnesses.

The health disparities that exist between native-born and foreign-born Blacks may be the result of selection bias, that is, the fact that healthier people and those with more resources are more likely to immigrate. This may also explain the lower rate of poverty among foreign-born Blacks and their higher rates of college attendance (Deal et al, 2014; Coles, 2016). Black immigrants, especially West Indians and Africans, are now significantly overrepresented among African Americans attending college. Many foreign-born Blacks seek to distance themselves from their native-born counterparts and are less likely to report being the target of racism or discrimination, which may also contribute to their health advantage. Nevertheless, the health advantage of black immigrants tends to decrease across generations for those in the US, a health pattern that supports the negative acculturation hypothesis (Williams and Sternthal, 2010).

African-American class disadvantage

Race and racist ideologies affect health in multiple ways and arenas, perhaps most powerfully through the perpetuation of black social class disadvantage and poverty. As Feagin and Bennefield have noted, for 336 years—85 percent of US history—slavery and segregation restricted opportunities for Blacks, while advantaging more than 20 generations of Whites with greater opportunities (Feagin and Bennefield, 2014). Social class disadvantage is recognized as the strongest predictor of sickness and early death, and it contributes to black-white racial disparities in health. Compared to Whites, African Americans are more likely to be unemployed and they earn significantly less. Data from the Bureau of Labor Statistics for the early months of 2016 show a national unemployment rate was 4.9 percent, but the rate of black unemployment (8.8 percent) was more than double that of white unemployment (4.3 percent). The median weekly earnings of African-American men and women who are employed full-time are considerably lower than that of their white counterparts. Black men earn 72.4 percent as much as white men ($624 per week compared to $931), and black women 83.4 percent as much as white women ($621 per week compared to $745).

More than a quarter of all African Americans live in poverty and more than one-half of all black children live in poor or low-income households. Poverty is inherently stressful—a major factor in many sicknesses—and it creates a host of living conditions and behaviors that are detrimental to health. Living in racially segregated neighborhoods is the result of an intersection of social class and racial inequality, and it exposes African Americans to high rates of crime, social disorder, and social isolation, all of which adversely affect health (Ross and Mirowsky, 2009). Such neighborhoods are also characterized by substandard schools and a lack of easy access to medical care, and they are often chosen as the sites for disposing toxic environmental waste. The adverse health effects of growing up in poverty are not completely mitigated by class mobility, as African Americans who grow up poor but attain middle-class status in adulthood still experience a health deficit (Vartanian and Houser, 2010).

Poverty is stressful and creates a set of social conditions that undermine health; it also signifies personal failure, especially in the context of a pervasive ideology of individual responsibility and upward mobility. The rags-to-riches life trajectory, where one succeeds through hard work and self-discipline, ignores racism and blocked opportunities, often leading people to blame themselves for failing to succeed (Kwate and Meyer, 2010). The least advantaged are often the most likely to assume responsibility for being poor, as they have fewer interactions with Whites and are less aware of how institutionalized racism affects their lives (Young, 2004). Most African Americans endorse the American Dream of success, and when they are unable to achieve it, it diminishes their life satisfaction, happiness, and mental health (Sellers and Neighbors, 2008).

African Americans have experienced considerable socioeconomic mobility since the civil rights movement; however, being middle class does not always ameliorate social class disadvantages or erase racial differences in health. One reason is that the middle class encompasses a broad range of incomes—anywhere from $40,000 to $100,000 (Gilbert, 2011)—and Blacks are less likely than Whites to have incomes at the top of that range. Even those with upper-middle-class positions often feel like racial tokens and face considerable pressure to prove themselves (Emirbayer and Desmond, 2015). But as Pattillo-McCoy has argued, the black and white middle classes remain "separate and unequal" in most respects, as African Americans are concentrated in lower-middle class jobs with less prestige and pay, and tend to live in "buffer" zones between inner cities and suburbs, marginal neighborhoods where they are exposed to more crime, poorer schools, and victimization (Pattillo-McCoy, 1999). Middle-class Blacks are also more likely than their white counterparts to have grown up in poverty, segregated neighborhoods, and fragile families, all of which predict poorer health in adulthood (Williams, 2012).

For these reasons, being in the middle class lessens but does not eliminate racial disparities in health (Hayward et al, 2000). One study pointed out that among college graduates between the ages of 25 and 74, 43.6% of Blacks describe themselves as having less than good health, compared to 26.7% of Whites (Bennefield, 2015). Black college-educated women (16.9 percent) are still more than twice as likely as white women (7 percent) to have diabetes (Hayward et al, 2000). Infant mortality rates for college-educated African Americans are more than twice as high for similarly educated white and Hispanic women (Williams, 2012). Black female college graduates, in fact, have higher rates of infant mortality than Hispanic and white women who have not completed high school.

Racialized social system and health

Middle-class African Americans have a better health profile than their lower-income and poor counterparts, but experience the health consequences of living in a racialized social system. The impact of race on health operates through the ideology of racism, which maintains that some groups are inherently inferior and superior to others. Racism is essentially a strategy for people who have power and privilege to maintain control over valuable resources (Lukachko et al, 2014). This helps explain why it persists, despite challenges to racist ideologies and policies. Although few people would argue that racism no longer exists or is inconsequential, there is substantial evidence that racial attitudes and policies have changed since the civil rights era. Racial discrimination has been declared illegal, affirmative action policies have led to more opportunities for African Americans, and efforts have been made to integrate schools and workplaces. Racial attitudes have changed significantly: more people support racial equality and public displays of racism are criticized.

These liberal racial attitudes and the penalization of overt racism, however, stand in sharp contrast to the persistence of racist thinking and outcomes. Scholars have argued that Jim Crow racism, with its emphasis on black inferiority and segregation, has simply been replaced by laissez-faire or liberal racism. In the latter, people voice support for racial equality, but defend the racial status quo and resist initiatives (for example, school busing, affirmative action) aimed at creating equality (Bobo et al, 1997). Despite significant progress, racism still operates powerfully at the ideological, cultural, and institutional levels in ways that disadvantage African Americans. Racism and racial stereotypes create a debilitating sense of stigma among African Americans (Link and Phelan, 2014), especially when their assumed inferiority seems confirmed by life circumstances. They also pave the way for and justify racial discrimination. The majority of African Americans report having been discriminated against, and studies find that even the perception of being discriminated against can adversely affect health, perhaps even more so for black women (Brown et al, 2003; Blodorn et al, 2016).

Studies frequently link the poor health outcomes of African Americans to inadequate access to medical care or their treatment by health care professionals. Doctors are overwhelmingly white, even more in the higher echelons of medicine, where decisions about physician training and practice and health care policy are made (Feagin and Bennefield, 2014). Physicians are not immune from embracing racial stereotypes: many experience significant social distance from their black patients and, regardless of the patient's social class background, they characterize them as less intelligent and less likely to follow medical advice—beliefs that undoubtedly affect clinical decisions (van Ryan and Burke, 2000). Encounters between white physicians and patients of color tend to be shorter and of lower quality, with less patient involvement and shared decision-making (Aronson et al, 2013). Overall, African Americans are less likely than Whites to have access to high quality care (Abraham, 1993), and they receive fewer medical procedures than Whites and generally poorer health care (Stepanikova, 2012; Xanthos et al, 2012).

Beyond these individual behaviors by physicians and health care professionals, however, is the more pervasive system of institutionalized racism that is less visible but even more powerful in reinforcing the dominant racial hierarchy and adversely affecting black health. For example, one national study examined how structural racism affected rates of myocardial infarction, a disease related to stress, among African Americans. They found that in states with the highest levels of structural racism, as measured by racial disparities in education, employment, judicial treatment, and political participation, African Americans had the highest rates of myocardial infarction (Lukachko et al, 2014). This resonates with the idea that most of the racism that impairs black health and longevity occurs outside the medical system and in everyday life experiences, where racial stereotypes and marginalization tacitly justify discrimination against African Americans.

For example, African-American men have historically been characterized as sexual predators who are prone to criminal behavior, black women as sexually promiscuous drains on the welfare system, and both as general menaces to society. These stereotypes have historically justified the economic and sexual exploitation of black men and women, and they continue to do so. Black men have experienced a long history of lynching and incarceration for allegedly raping white women, but also for offenses as minor as petty theft. This criminalization of African-American men was historically motivated by efforts to place them in prison work camps or to keep them from voting (Holloway, 2014). Black men are still characterized as criminally inclined, and currently constitute such a significant proportion of the incarcerated population that it has become a major political and social issue. They are disproportionately stopped, harassed, and arrested by law enforcement officers: by the age of 30 black men have a 20 percent risk of being incarcerated, compared to 3 percent for white men (Massoglia, 2008b).

Racial stereotypes of African-American men as criminals have led to a recent spate of highly publicized cases of police officers beating or shooting unarmed men to death over minor offenses. This treatment is hardly new, but now is more easily captured by videos and widely distributed via social media, leading to massive protests and futile calls for justice. In one case, the black male was 12-year-old Tamir Rice, who was playing with a toy gun in a park across the street from his home. Tamir was killed by a police officer who discharged his weapon within seconds of arriving at the scene, an incident that sent a chilling message to African-American parents about the value of their children. Research and investigations by the Department of Justice document rampant racism in many large police departments. Nicole Gonzalez van Cleue, a professor who once worked as a court clerk in Chicago, witnessed first-hand how racism affects the arrest and sentencing of African Americans. She pointed out that collusion between judges and police officers in convicting African-American men is common. It includes not only blatant perjury in the testimony of police officers, but a culture where black men are described as "dogs" and their speech patterns, ethnic names, and manner of dressing are openly mocked. Even officers who may not agree with such conduct are silenced by the threat of job loss, or worse (van Cleue, 2016).

African-American women are not exempt from violence at the hands of police officers over minor offenses or incarceration. On July 3, 2015, Sandra Bland, a 28-year-old black women, was found hanged in her jail cell in Waller County, Texas after being arrested for a minor traffic offense. Although her death was ruled a suicide, it raised suspicions and reinforced the lack of value law enforcement officials place on black lives. Rape was historically and continues to be used as a weapon to control black women. An Oklahoma police officer was recently convicted of 18 counts of first-degree rape and other forms of sexual victimization against low-income black women in the neighborhood he was assigned to patrol. The police officer randomly stopped, searched, and assaulted these women, threatening to arrest and imprison them for drugs or other crimes if they reported the rape. One arrested black woman was hospitalized and handcuffed to her hospital bed at the time of the assault. Another, a 17-year-old black teenager, was raped by the officer on her mother's front porch. The devastating effect of this sexual terrorism can be heard in her words: "Every time I see the police, I don't even know what do to. I don't ever go outside, and when I do I'm terrified." Some comfort might be derived from thinking these were the acts of one rogue officer, but statistics reveal that this is not the case (Murphy, 2016).

Low-income African Americans often seem to bear the brunt of the racialized social system, but racism transcends class boundaries. In 2015, nine black churchgoers in South Carolina lost their lives in a racially inspired shooting. Other cases abound—a black college professor at an elite university arrested on his own porch because he was suspected of breaking and entering, a prominent black tennis player wrestled to the ground by an off-duty police officer due to mistaken identity, the stigmatizing of Blacks who worked hard to achieve success as tokens of affirmative action, and the recent boycott by African-American celebrities of a major awards show that failed to nominate a single person of color. Michelle Obama, First Lady in the US, recently shared how she had been caricatured in the media as a terrorist, referred to as "Obama's baby Momma," and described as perhaps "too angry, too loud, and too emasculating" for her role. The notion of black inferiority is evident in the recent comments of some Supreme Court justices as they heard arguments over a case of affirmation action. One questioned whether racial diversity in fields like science and technology really mattered, and another opined that African Americans might perform better in second-tier schools.

Racism and racial inequality perpetuate the gap in quality of life between Blacks and Whites. Bonilla-Silva has recently proposed that we live with a "racial grammar" that normalizes whiteness—white beliefs, white behaviors, white cultural standards—in ways that reinforce white supremacy in invisible but powerful ways (Bonilla-Silva, 2012). One implication of this is the overall gap in the quality of life for Blacks and Whites. The National Urban League's Equality Index provides an annual comparison across five categories (social justice, health, economy, education, and civic engagement), providing a comprehensive picture of racial disparities in wellbeing. In 2015 African Americans scored 72.2, which means the quality of these conditions for them was less than 75 percent of that for Whites (Coles, 2016). These racial gaps in quality of life conditions help explain why social class alone falls short of explaining black-white health disparities. African Americans across the social class spectrum have worse health than Whites.

Conclusion

Racism and discrimination are chronic stressors for African Americans. Racism manifests itself in widely accepted racial stereotypes about black people that reinforce racist behaviors and ideologies, and it is institutionalized in the practices and policies of social institutions ranging from governments and schools, from medical settings to police departments.

The persistence of racism and racial inequality more than 50 years after the passage of civil rights policies creates an environment of chronic stress for African Americans, perhaps made even more frustrating in a nation that has elected its first black president. For many, the election of an African-American president signified notable racial progress, even an evolving post-racial society. Yet for many Whites it sparked deep concerns about a new racial order and an almost frenzied opposition to every act initiated by the President, perhaps none more than health care reform. Rather than working to unify the nation and improve the lives of Americans through negotiation and compromise across political lines, one leader of the Republican party, Senator Mitch McConnell, expressed the sentiment of many conservatives when he declared that his top political priority was to deny President Obama a second term in office.

Growing economic inequality and fewer opportunities for class mobility have led many Whites to fear that they are losing ground to racial minorities and immigrants, and some have become more receptive to openly racist political messages. At the same time black frustration over continuing racism and exclusion has increased, sharpening racial tensions and divisions and sparking a new wave of social protest across the nation. In 1995, many African Americans participated in the Million Man March that called on black men to step up to the responsibilities of fatherhood and family life, and become more active in improving the quality of life for those in black communities. A second march, 20 years later, entitled "Justice or Else," had a distinctively different tone. Leaders of the 2015 march argued that justice was the birthright of every human being, and contended:

> The widespread death, rising racism, mob attacks and police brutality on Blacks, coupled with economic deprivation and stark poverty, requires that something must be immediately done to address and correct the situation.

Black Lives Matter, a group of mostly young, loosely organized African-American activists and their allies, have also taken up the call for social justice. They are demanding an end to police violence but also the more pervasive racialized environment where racial minorities are excluded, neglected, and made invisible while whiteness is prominently depicted or displayed. Many Americans agree that change is needed: in 2015, 60 percent of Americans believed that the nation needed to continue to make changes that assure equal rights and opportunities for Blacks. African Americans (85 percent) were more likely to express that opinion than white Americans (53 percent); still this represents a notable increase in the number of Whites (39 percent) who felt that way just a year ago (Drake, 2016).

TWO

Sickness in slavery and freedom

The health deficit that exists among African Americans and is perpetuated by a racialized social system can more broadly be understood by placing it within historical context, especially the centuries of slavery and racial segregation that black people endured. Most Africans were brought to the US involuntarily, enslaved, exposed to dismal diets and living conditions, and subjected to brutal punishment and mechanisms of social control. These harsh conditions contributed to the health maladies that were common among most immigrants to the New World, such as the widespread exposure to infectious diseases that usually could not be reliably controlled by medical interventions.

Emancipation proved an even greater health disaster for the formerly enslaved, as the freed men and women lost whatever value they previously held as the property of slave owners and entered a society that had made few provisions for the transition of more than four million people from slavery to freedom. The question of whether African Americans would be integrated into the US population was not decided until 1896, when the Supreme Court legalized racial segregation with a "separate but equal" doctrine. Racial segregation remained legal until the civil rights movement of the 1960s, and made it difficult for African Americans to obtain adequate medical care, an issue compounded by the fact that Blacks had at best restricted access to medical education.

The ascendancy of modern scientific medicine, already underway by the mid-1800s, also had significant consequences for African Americans. Enslaved black people were often used for medical experimentation and, once slavery was abolished, the medical profession promoted theories of black inferiority through a form of scientific racism that argued the health issues facing African Americans were due to their inherent moral, biological, and cultural deficiencies. For the bulk of the 20th century a racially-based dual health care system offered African Americans substandard care, often in overcrowded segregated hospital wards.

Notable histories on the rise of modern scientific medicine rarely include much about black health care during or after slavery, or the struggle of African Americans to obtain health care and become health care professionals. This chapter helps write that history into the story of the US health care system. I start with an examination of health and health issues among enslaved black Africans in colonial America, and then explore how emancipation affected their health and access to medical care. I contend that the health deficit of African Americans today, along with some of their health behaviors and decisions, are deeply rooted in a medical care system that promoted scientific racism, used African Americans for medical experiments, denied Blacks adequate medical care, and excluded them from the practice of medicine. This chapter also highlights the agency of African Americans in pursuing justice in medical care.

Health of black Africans in early America

The health and health care of the black Africans brought to what later became America is best understood within the broader context of colonial life in the 1600s. Life for most of the early colonists was characterized by a perilous journey of immigration from Europe to the New World and the hardships of constructing life on unsettled frontiers. Many early English immigrants were motivated by the hope of greater religious freedom, but were also escaping a rapidly developing industrial economy in Europe, which displaced workers and created dire living conditions. Still, the first White settlers in the New World faced almost insurmountable obstacles to survival, such as malnutrition, starvation, and sickness (Shryock, 1966). The summers brought high rates of diphtheria, smallpox, and malaria—especially as communities grew in size—and deaths from respiratory illnesses were common in the winter. Even in sparsely settled areas, sicknesses were prolific and a constant source of concern; indeed, the diaries and writings of early colonists are filled with concerns about health and healing (Savitt, 1978, 2005). Infectious diseases and an absence of effective medical care made sickness, infant and maternal mortality, and early death common.

Black Africans were among the earliest settlers to come to North America from abroad: 20 enslaved Blacks were brought to the shores of Jamestown, Virginia in 1619. Slavery already existed in Spain and England, but in the colonies it took most of the 17th century to clearly define chattel slavery, clarify the legal status of enslaved Blacks, and have their treatment codified into law (Byrd and Clayton, 2000). Once complete, that process had instituted perpetual and hereditary servitude, stripped enslaved people of rights over their person or property, and defined them as property. So in addition to being exposed to the diseases prevalent among Whites, the health of enslaved Blacks was further jeopardized by their racial status. As Byrd and Clayton (2000) have explained, slaves entered North America with substantial health deficits, often stemming from being captured, held in slave castles, surviving the Middle Passage, and in some cases enduring up to a three-year "breaking in" process in the New World. Conservative estimates are that the mortality rate among Blacks—from their sale or capture in Africa to their entry into slavery—was about 50 percent, though some argue it was much higher.

Slavery thrived for more than two-and-a-half centuries in the United States, and the unpaid labor of slaves played a crucial role in building the wealth of the nation (Baptist, 2014). But it also contributed inestimably to poor health and the dismal living conditions of black people. Beyond the common travails of sickness experienced by all early Americans, the health of slaves was jeopardized further by poor housing, lack of sanitation, and work schedules that often required them to work from dawn to dusk practically every day of the year. Slave quarters were typically filthy, often infested with huge numbers of pests and parasites, and enslaved Blacks were given very little time or resources for bathing, or washing their hair, clothing, or beds (Savitt, 1978; Byrd and Clayton, 2000). Nearly all children and many adults lacked shoes or sufficient clothing. It was not uncommon for younger children to be naked (Savitt, 1978) and field workers so scantily clad that they tried to hide when strangers approached (Owens, 1976). Cultivating crops like tobacco, rice, and sugar cane had especially adverse health consequences, and the diets of slaves, consisting largely of pork, corn, and cornmeal, contributed to poor health (Savitt, 1978). Eating soured and spoiled food was a constant source of sickness, especially among Blacks owned by small slave owners with only a few slaves.

Historians have documented that infectious diseases like body lice, ringworm, and bedbugs were especially common among slaves, as were more life-threatening respiratory illnesses. Colds, flu, diarrhea, and pneumonia were prolific sources of sickness and death, and malarial fevers (for example, typhoid, yellow, and scarlet) were especially dreaded and likely to lead to death (Owens, 1976). Sexually transmitted diseases (STDs) were prevalent among the poor regardless of race, but more so among enslaved Africans. Casual sexual activity among slaves was often encouraged, as it increased fertility and weakened family ties. Byrd and Clayton reported that slave quarters were incubators for STDs, especially syphilis, which was sometimes congenital. The standard treatment of STDs was costly, relatively ineffective, and unavailable to the poor, especially enslaved Blacks.

Pregnancy and childbirth were high-risk ventures for most women during the colonial era, as rates of maternal and infant mortality were high. This was compounded for black women, who were often coerced into sexual liaisons and expected to produce babies. The extent to which slave owners participated in the deliberate breeding of slaves has been a topic of some debate; however, there is much evidence that the practice was common, especially after the importation of slaves was officially banned in the early 1800s. In his historical research using slave records, Stampp found numerous references to the profitability of slave breeding and descriptions of women as "good breeders" (Stampp, 1956). Research by Byrd and Clayton agrees. They write:

> Slave women were encouraged, cajoled, and coerced by their owners to become pregnant. For not complying, some were whipped or sold. Some female slaves were purchased specifically for breeding. Women were often forced to engage in intercourse with strange men and males to whom they were not attracted. (Byrd and Clayton, 2000: 282)

Black children were potentially important sources of labor and capital for slave owners, and there was some concern over their high rates of death. Slave owners sometimes worried about high rates of miscarriage among their female slaves, fearing that they were deliberately aborting their pregnancies. But even those who managed full-term pregnancies had high rates of stillbirth, low birth weight infants, and infant mortality, likely due to the work patterns, nutrition, and the nursing practices of enslaved women. The high rate of infant death also resulted from lockjaw, due to poisonous breast milk from mothers. Some felt babies should be deprived of that milk, and came up with various ways to drain women's breasts, including the use of puppies (Long, 2012). Malnutrition was common among black children, and they seemed predisposed to diarrhea and respiratory illnesses. It was not uncommon for black children to be killed by rats or to die from worm infestations or diseases carried by fleas and insects (Byrd and Clayton, 2000).

The harsh punishment endured by black slaves created another source of sickness, injury, and death (Baptist, 2014). While laws forbade certain types of punishment for white indentured servants, such laws were not extended to enslaved Blacks. Whippings and food deprivation were common forms of punishment meted out to the poor and indentured servants but, as many have pointed out, mutilation, castration, nose-splitting, branding, crippling, and burning alive was almost exclusively reserved as punishments for those held in chattel slavery (Bankole, 1998; Byrd and Clayton, 2000; Baptist, 2014). A woman formerly enslaved in Louisiana, Mary Reynolds, said:

> Slavery was the worst days that ever seed in the world. They was things past tellin', but I got the scars on my old body to show to this day. I seed worse than happened to me. (Bankole, 1998: 5)

Although there was some debate over whether keeping slaves healthy or working them to death and replacing them was the most profitable, the former strategy seemed to prevail as slavery became more institutionalized and the importation of more slaves was prohibited. The prosperity of slave owners depended on the productive labor of slaves, even more so as the average price of a slave who worked in the field rose from $200 in 1793 to $1,000 in 1850 (Morais, 1968). While the growing value of slaves might have led to better treatment, the proliferation of slave revolts led to harsher penalties during the 1800s.

The extraordinary expansion of the nation's territory during the early through late 1800s made slavery even more vital to the economy; in fact, the policies of President Andrew Jackson included subjugating black people to permanent slavery and dispossessing Native Americans of their land to accommodate the expansion. The slave population grew from 1,771,656 in 1820 to 4,441,830 by the start of the Civil War, as enslaved Blacks were sent to western and southwest territories where they were subjected to the "most brutal and heavy work imaginable"—for example, land clearance, swamp drainage, tree removal, and preparing virgin land for crops like cotton, sugar cane, and rice (Byrd and Clayton, 2000). The expansion of slavery into these new areas had a devastating impact on black families, separating husbands from wives and parents from children, and contributed immensely to the black health deficit. With a more than doubling of the enslaved population, however, unrest over slavery was growing, and it was abolished in a few states. Thus, the free black population began to gradually expand.

Medical care in early America

Families were the center of social and economic life in early America and the arena in which most medical care was dispensed. From the 1600s through the late 18th century, tending the sick took place in the domestic arena and was typically the responsibility of women. Little was known about the etiology of sickness, though it was widely believed that immorality and sin predisposed people to sickness and healing came through prayer, repentance, and medical interventions. For the latter, families kept on hand a stock of healing remedies passed on from earlier generations or gleaned from medical manuals. It was not uncommon for the home medicine chest to contain a wide array of medicines and medical devices—for example, calomel, castor oil, ipecac, jalap, opium camphor, and quinine were commonly stocked in homes, along with lancets, spatulas, and blister powders (Savitt, 1978).

Enslaved Blacks often drew on ancient African healing traditions such as herbs, roots, and conjuring. Although these strategies were often seen as primitive and of little medicinal value, Morais (1968) has argued that there were very few noticeable differences between the healing strategies of enslaved Africans and Whites. For both, treatment of illness occurred within the family, although the labor demands of slaves curtailed the time they were given to tend to the sick. For the most part, Blacks and Whites relied heavily on spiritual interpretations of illness and herbs, charms, plants, and minerals for healing. Black women were especially called on as midwives and for providing folk cures, and historians have found some instances in which enslaved Blacks were emancipated or given special privileges because of their healing abilities (Savitt, 1978, 2005; Byrd and Clayton, 2000).

Black women in the South, called "grannies" or "mormers," often provided nursing care to the sick (Banks, 2011). Some Blacks with notable healing skills were called on to heal Whites, but they faced considerable risk when doing so. Slave owners lived in constant fear of being harmed or poisoned by slaves, and when the efforts of slaves to effect healing were unsuccessful or resulted in the death of the patient, even those slaves with good intentions could face dire consequences. Colonial states prohibited slaves from administering medicine to anyone—black or white—without the explicit approval of their masters, and passed laws authorizing the death penalty in such cases. These laws, undoubtedly, made the practice of medicine a risky enterprise for enslaved black people, but did not end it. Between 1731 and 1812 black practitioners across the US, but especially in the South, created a slave health subsystem of various healers, including conjurers, root doctors, and others drawing on African traditions (Byrd and Clayton, 2000).

Slave owners were responsible for the health care of their slaves and authorized treatments at their own discretion. Claiming sickness could be risky for slaves, however, as it could result in punishment for malingering or being forced to accept whatever medical remedy they were offered (Long, 2012). One white physician in Georgia noted:

> The negro is prone to dissemble and feign disease; probably no race of human beings feign themselves ill so frequently, and are so incapable of concealing their duplicity. (Savitt, 1978: 163)

Slave owners had to balance concern over malingering slaves with the cost of losing human chattel or having their diseases spread to their own families, and they drew on a variety of people to help manage sickness among slaves. Slave owners' wives or overseers were often given that responsibility, and some larger plantations set up slave hospitals. In severe cases of illness they called upon white doctors to treat their patients, as many claimed to have special knowledge about black diseases. Still, they could not ignore the healing abilities of many Blacks—enslaved and free—or the confidence that slaves often had in such healers. Slaves were often fearful of the medicines administered by their white owners, and in many cases were more responsive to the treatment of black healers. Slaves with known healing abilities, sometimes from nearby plantations, were often called on with favorable results (Owens, 1976).

As the population expanded with successive waves of European immigration and the steady importation of slaves, so did the array of healers and healing strategies that were practiced. In *The social transformation of American medicine*, Paul Starr noted that in pre-industrial America there were three dominant practitioners, all fairly equal in status: physicians, domestic healers, and lay healers (for example, bonesetters, midwives, botanists, etc) (Starr, 1982: 32). There was little agreement on either the cause or proper treatment of illness and the lack of a medical infrastructure made home care popular. Medical training was varied; nearly anyone who wanted to could practice medicine, and many did. By the late 1700s there were at least 4,000 medical practitioners, about 400 of whom had medical training—which ranged from having studied in Europe at a prestigious medical school to having completed a relatively short apprenticeship in the US. The elite of the profession were "gentlemen" who refused to work with their hands, while those who learned medicine through an apprenticeship often used healing strategies as lethal as the disease, for example, bleeding, purging, and blistering.

Race and racism in medicine

As black slavery expanded and became more institutionalized, early theories of Africans as innately inferior to white Europeans also spread and influenced the practice and development of medicine, aiding in the exploitation of black people for economic gain. In medicine, black people were often compared with apes, and thus seen as non-human, unintelligent, and uncivilized. It was common to explain this with pseudo-scientific theories, such as the "great chain of being," which argued that there was a progression from groups that were simple and animalistic to those who were advanced human beings. Blacks, of course, fell into the former group and were often subjected to tours that focused on their physical differences as proof of their less than human status. The case of Saartjie Baartman, a member of the Kung tribe of Bushmen of South Africa, is one of the best known examples. Saartjie was considered beautiful by her people, a group known as the Hottentots, but by Whites an example of one of the lowest forms of humanity (Byrd and Clayton, 2000).

Medical science eagerly embraced and advanced racist ideologies, which were uncritically accepted by most physicians. The consensus in the medical community was that black people were mentally and medically inferior to Whites, and that the "Negro race ... is a distinct species with separate origin from Caucasians" (Savitt, 1978: 8). Medical science documented the peculiarities of black people (for example, large breasts and penises, unbridled sexuality, strong body odors, strong tolerance for pain) and categorized certain diseases, such as chronic leprosy, locked jaw, and difficult parturition, as black diseases. Benjamin Rush, perhaps the most famous physician of the colonial era and an anti-slavery activist, advanced theories that contributed to scientific racism. Rush argued that the black skin, facial features, body odor, relative insensitivity to pain, and notorious sexuality of black people were due to a congenital, chronic form of leprosy.

Medical theories on racial differences were prolific, and usually framed in ways supportive of slavery and black inferiority. For example, studies pointed out that black people had lower rates of lunacy or mental illness—a fact attributed to their being simple and unthinking beings who had few worries because they were clothed and fed by others. Data collected for the 1840 federal census were used to claim that Blacks who were free were eleven times more likely than those who were enslaved to suffer from mental deficiencies, just one indicator of the perils of freedom for Blacks. William Weaver, a Southerner who was superintendent of the census, argued: "The African is incapable of self-care and sinks into lunacy under the burden of freedom. It is a mercy to give him guardianship and protection from mental death" (quoted in Morais, 1968: 32). Such knowledge prevailed, despite critics of the report who noted that some northern towns reported as having mentally ill Blacks actually had no black population at all. Biological determinism was central to the American worldview and embraced by scientific medicine; historians have noted that "this was not a fringe movement or the product of some group of ignorant, poorly educated extremists" (Byrd and Clayton, 2000: 248).

Despite this emphasis on racial differences in sicknesses which, presumably, would suggest the need for racially specific medical interventions, enslaved and freed African Americans—along with poor people in general—were widely used in medical experiments. Slave owners dosed their slaves with medical remedies to test their effectiveness, and Thomas Jefferson—a slave owner and founding father of the nation—tested vaccines using slaves (Downs, 2012). Slaves were especially used to demonstrate medical techniques and to test surgical procedures in an era when surgery was considered a death sentence. Medical schools and hospitals, in fact, boasted of having an abundance of "medical material" for their work (Savitt, 1978). Medical doctors and their students also disinterred bodies from pauper and black cemeteries, although the practice was illegal. J. Marion Sims, often called the father of gynecology, perfected his vaginal surgery techniques almost entirely on enslaved black women, often without anesthesia. In a few cases he conducted 20-30 surgeries on a single patient to correct the failures and mistakes of previous surgeries. Although some argued that Blacks were relatively insensitive to pain, in his clinical notes on one case of surgery on an enslaved black woman, Sims recorded: "Lucy's agony was extreme. She was much prostrated and I thought she was going to die.... It took Lucy two or three months to recover entirely from the effects of the operation" (Bankole, 1998: 19).

Emancipation: a crisis of sickness and death

Historians and other scholars have documented the dramatic surge in disease, sickness, and death among the newly freed slaves that began during the Civil War and lasted through the early decades of the 20th century. Some estimate that as many as 25 percent of the black population died of sickness during the War and the early years of freedom (Smith, 1995). An in-depth analysis has been provided by Jim Downs' in *Sick from freedom: African-American illness and suffering during the Civil War and reconstruction*. Downs pointed out that contagious infections and diseases often caused more death during war than combat, and the Civil War was no exception. Overcrowding, unsanitary living conditions in army camps, insufficient resources, and the inability of medicine to control epidemics resulted in the death of thousands of soldiers from dysentery, pneumonia, smallpox, and measles. But those conditions took an even greater toll on the more than four million slaves who were liberated in a nation that was ill-equipped to handle their transition to freedom.

Thousands of slaves joined the Union Army, many motivated by the Militia Act of 1862. It declared that every enslaved man or boy who enlisted—if their masters were disloyal to the Union—would be freed, along with his mother and children (Long, 2012). Other slaves made the perilous journey to Union military camps seeking refuge, in some cases only to be sent back as violators of the Fugitive Slave Act. In other cases, they were declared "contraband of war," confiscated as animals, and put to work performing manual labor. Living in military camps not only exposed them to diseases but confined them to makeshift communities where the living conditions were abysmal and food shortages and starvation common. Their initial dislocation was often compounded by being moved from camp to camp, with little concern for those who were sick or emaciated.

The War devastated the agricultural economy of the South, leading to high rates of poverty, famine, and poor health. Southern states could scarcely provide health care and other assistance for their white citizens and, as Beardsley has argued, they had practically no incentive to provide help to African Americans (Beardsley, 1990). Debate raged among politicians over whether the states or the federal government should assume responsibility for providing medical care for former slaves. The federal government finally responded by establishing a Medical Division of the Freedmen's Bureau, which built hospitals and almshouses and staffed them with hundreds of health care workers. Such facilities, however, fell far short of providing health care to the newly freed slaves, whose poor health was explained as indicative of their inferiority. The collection of data by the federal government supported theories of innate black health inferiority, as it found that by the late 19th century Blacks had higher rates of sickness than Whites and shorter life spans. At this time, the life span for Whites was 50 compared to 30-32 for black men an 34 for black women (Byrd and Clayton, 2000), further evidence of greater black vulnerability to poor health and early death. Moreover, the mission of the Medical Division was to create a healthy labor force, and concern that providing health care services to black people would foster dependency led to limited funding and resources (Downs, 2012).

The health and mortality crisis resulting from emancipation and the absence of adequate policies to aid formerly enslaved Blacks in adapting to freedom continued throughout the early decades of the 20th century. The problem was exacerbated as African Americans left rural areas and plantations and made their way into southern urban areas. As Long has explained:

> The newly arrived African Americans faced an immediate housing and employment shortage. The inadequate housing procured by many was crowded, ill ventilated, and bereft of a sanitary water supply or functioning sewage system. These problems, combined with poverty and unemployment, made for the ideal conditions for the spread of epidemic diseases such as smallpox, cholera, and yellow fever. (Long, 2012: 102)

Some southern states that once had provided a modicum of health care for the poor now insisted that those services were for citizens only, which excluded African Americans. Smallpox, cholera, and yellow fever took a devastating toll on Blacks, most of whom did not receive (and sometimes simply refused) the vaccines that were available. Black fertility rates declined sharply between 1867 and 1935, attributed mainly to sexually transmitted diseases, poor diets, and unsanitary living and birthing conditions (Beardsley, 1990). Poor health and high rates of death among African Americans reinforced the "theory of racial degeneracy"—a belief widely held by politicians, doctors, and the public that slavery had a civilizing impact on black people, but with freedom they were reverting to their native savagery (Summers, 2014). Some public health doctors argued that improved environmental conditions would help, but most held that Blacks suffered due to their "inherent shiftlessness, low intelligence, and love of carnal pleasure" (Beardsley, 1990: 124).

Articles in the *Journal of the American Medical Association* in the early decades of the 20th century examining the health plight of "the negro" emphasized that the abolition of slavery had resulted in high rates of insanity, consumption, syphilis, and immorality among black people. In a 1900 address before the Tri-State Medical Society of Virginia and the Carolinas, Dr Barringer argued that Blacks were reverting to savagery so rapidly that "unless a brake is placed on ontogeny of this savage, the South will be uninhabitable for whites." A revisionist perspective on the harsh realities of slavery cast it as a paternalistic system in which Blacks were well-cared for. An article by Dr Murrell argued that as a "valuable form of energy," enslaved Blacks received the best of housing, nutrition, and clothing in order to maximize their labor potential, and then—overlooking the impact of the absence of those basic resources necessary for survival—he explained that with abolition "morality [became] a joke among these people." According to another doctor:

> Freedom removed all hygienic restraints and they [Blacks] were no longer obedient to the inexorable laws of health, plunging into all sorts of excesses and vices, and having apparently little control over their appetites and passions. (Powell, 1896: 1186)

Others linked the lack of mortality to the development of the brain. A short article in the *Journal of the American Medical Association* noted:

> The lower mental faculties of the negro, such as smell, sight, handicraftmanship, body-sense and melody, are well developed, but in the higher faculties, self-control, will power, ethical and aesthetic senses, and reason, the negro falls considerably behind the Caucasian. (*Journal of the American Medical Association*, 1906)

Many believed Blacks were on the verge of racial extinction, and there were few efforts to reverse that trend. The presumed biological inferiority of black people was used as evidence of the ill-effects of miscegenation. In the mid-1800s the federal census counted the number of mulattoes in the slave population with the goal of examining the mental and health consequences of being interracial. Census data revealed white ancestry was common among slaves—about 20 percent of slaves in some states were mulattoes and 30 percent of free Blacks were mulattoes, leaving one historian to muse that slavery was getting "whiter and whiter" (Humphreys, 2008). Miscegenation became the focus of the medical community. In 1907, the Tennessee State Medical Association offered a medical report that pointed out:

> It is principally the yellow Negro that shows the enormous death-rate from tuberculosis today. In all cases, wherever we find a hybrid race, we find a race which has not the stamina, physical, moral or mental, of either of the races in the mixture. (quoted in Smith, 1999: 22)

Throughout the first half of the 20th century, doctors and medical scientists continued to argue that black people had an inherited immunity to certain diseases, such as malaria, influenza, and the mumps, and a propensity towards others, such as tuberculosis (Oppenheimer, 2001). Most embraced the "black pest thesis," referring to black people as vectors for diseases that could infect white people. These medical theories resonated with the 1896 US Supreme Court decision legalizing racial segregation and provided the foundation for the segregated medical system.

The rise of the dual health care system

The modernization of the American health care system emerged amid emancipation and a rapidly industrializing economy. By modernization is meant the rise of scientific medicine and of professional dominance by allopathic physicians, their power garnered largely from advances in medical knowledge and political lobbying.

As late as 1850, allopathic or "regular physicians" struggled for control over the health care system but remained "weak, divided, insecure in its status and its income, [and] unable to control entry into practice or raise the standard of medical education" (Starr, 1982: 7-8). But the final decades of that century proved transformative for them as the germ theory of sickness became the basis for scientific medicine. The rise of scientific medicine and the power and authority of physicians resonated with the turn of the century emphasis of modernization, professionalization, and science. Membership in the American Medical Association (AMA), which was founded in 1846, soared in the last decades of the century, as it became the best-funded and most powerful lobby in US. Through these efforts, physicians lobbied for and received a virtual monopoly on the right to practice medicine (Freidson, 1970).

The modernization of medical care and the rise of scientific medicine led to a vast expansion of the health care industry and a standardization and improvement in medical care. Providing medical care was no longer the responsibility of the family but was transferred to doctors and hospitals. In 1873 there were fewer than 200 hospitals in the US, but by 1920 there were more than 6,000 (Starr, 1982). The separate but equal doctrine established in 1896 led to the creation of a dual health care system based on race. Southern states constructed their entire hospital system on the doctrine of racial separation, and African-American patients in the North also often received care in racially segregated facilities (Quadagno, 2000). The years between 1832 through 1965 marked the height of segregation in the field of medicine. Black patients usually found themselves in segregated waiting rooms in doctors' offices and medical facilities, where they often had to wait until white patients were served before receiving treatment. As one African-American female recalled:

> I remember when I was a teen I had to help my grandmom go for care at Greenville General. She had cancer. We had to wait in a horrible small room for black patients in the basement. We'd get there by 9:00, and we often didn't return until 5:30. The local mortician provided the transportation to the hospital. The understanding was that the transportation was free, but he would get the body. It wasn't a bad experience. It was the way it was. (quoted in Smith, 1999: 10)

Access to hospital care was scarce for black patients during the early 20th century. Most hospitals did not accept African Americans, and those that did usually relegated them to segregated wards that were dilapidated and overcrowded. Of the 127 Veteran Administration hospitals that existed in 1947, 24 of them had separate wards for black patients and another 19 admitted Blacks only for emergency treatments (Shea and Fullilove, 1985). In 1930, only 225 of the nation's 7,259 hospital beds were reserved for black patients (Morais, 1968). Black patients sometimes died after being taken to a hospital where all the "black beds" were taken, even if some "white beds" were still empty. African-American doctors and their supporters, however, managed to establish at least one black hospital in nearly every southern state. The most famous was the Tuskegee Institute Hospital and Nurses Training

School founded in Alabama in 1892, which, after the First World War, became the center of care for over 300,000 black veterans in the South (Watson, 1999). Still, having the hospital staffed by black health care professionals was the result of a prolonged battle between white supremacists and black physicians and their supporters.

African-American health care workers

African Americans interested in providing medical care also found themselves relegated to the margins of medicine. Although those who had traditionally practiced spiritual and folk healing were now stigmatized as superstitious or quacks, there were limited opportunities for Blacks who wanted to study scientific medicine to attend medical schools. Some African Americans had managed to obtain formal medical training in the 1800s, and by 1890 there were 909 black male doctors (Hine and Thompson, 1998). Between 1848 and 1860, the closing decades of slavery, five medical schools admitted black students: Bowdoin, Harvard, Dartmouth, Western Homeopathic College, and the New England Female Medical College (Watson, 1999). After the abolition of slavery, several black medical schools were established, including Howard University Medical School and Meharry Medical College. Many white people were amused at the notion that African Americans could become physicians, as the two statuses seemed so incongruous. Long (2012) noted that caricatures of black doctors were common in the media, such as an 1899 publication titled *The medicine man – A coon song*.

Although women were being driven from the field of medicine, a few managed to get formal medical training. In 1864 Rebecca Lee graduated from the New England Female Medical College in Boston and became the first black woman to earn a medical degree. Most black women who completed medical school held little hope of practicing in the US and acquired medical training in order to become missionaries and use their training to work in poor nations, especially Africa (Watson, 1999). Black women, especially in southern states, continued to be heavily involved in midwifery, which they considered an extremely prestigious occupation. In the early 1920s southern states hired public health nurses to oversee midwives, to make sure they were registered, wore proper clothing, and met other health-related requirements. But white physicians increasingly criticized the role of women in delivering babies. In 1925, a prominent physician described the black midwife as "filthy and ignorant and not far removed from the jungles of Africa, laden with its atmosphere of weird superstitions and voodooism" (Smith, 1995: 125).

In the early decades of the 20th century African-American medical students continued to face formidable barriers in acquiring a medical education and practicing medicine. One problem was that most of the black medical schools founded in the post-slavery era were closed by the early 20th century, as they were unable to meet the educational standards set forth in the Flexner Report on medical education. The Flexner Report reinforced the racial divide in medicine and the marginalization and shortage of African-American doctors. The section of the report entitled "The medical education of the negro" endorsed training of some black doctors, "if the negro can be brought to feel a sharp responsibility for the physical integrity of his people." It argued that black doctors should be trained mostly in preventive medicine, rather than fields like surgery, and should be trained to "humbly" serve black people as "sanitarians" (Long, 2012: 58). Flexner focused on the public health function of black doctors, noting that Whites needed a barrier from the diseases and infections that were common among African Americans (Summers, 2014).

Few African Americans were able to enter medical schools. Between 1920 and 1964, only 2-3 percent of students entering medical schools (mostly Howard or Meharry) were Blacks. Once they completed medical school black doctors found it difficult to obtain the residencies or internships they needed to complete their training. In 1927, for example, only 21 of the 1,696 hospitals in the nation employed black interns, and of them, 14 treated only black patients (Blount, 1984). Most black doctors were unable to train in the most prestigious medical specialties and were concentrated in fields such as family medicine and pediatrics. Sonnie Wellington Hereford, who was trained at Meharry in the 1950s and practiced medicine in Alabama, described the segregated hospital this way:

> The Colored Wing had one large room that served as our emergency room, delivery room, and operating room—what we called the ER, DR, and OR. The hallways could accommodate another ten or twelve beds; the administration did not mind having people lying out in the hall so long as nobody tried to go over to the other side. (Hereford, 2011: 58)

Racial codes governed everything from minor issues (for example, clerks refused to put "Mr" or "Mrs" on black patients' records) to access to facilities and behavior. Dr Hereford pointed out: "We were not permitted to eat at staff meetings. We were not permitted to dictate our records on the hospital Dictaphone. We were not permitted to administer anesthesia. We had to watch ourselves every step of the way … to be a perfect gentleman every minute."

Another factor restricting the professional development of black doctors was their inability to join the AMA. Although it claimed to have no racial restrictions on admission—and it did have some black members—only doctors who were members of the local medical society could join. But many of these local medical societies, especially those in the South, did not admit African-American doctors. This marginalized black doctors, since membership was linked to hospital privileges, access to state licensing bodies, forming supportive networks, and participation at conferences where new research was presented (Baker et al, 2008).

African-American physicians fought for membership in the AMA but also formed their own state and local medical societies, perhaps most notably in 1895 establishing the National Medical Association. They also founded the *Journal of the National Medical Association* and published numerous articles that challenged the claims by white physicians and scientists that poor health among African Americans was the result of biological inferiority. They led the charge in attributing the poor health of African Americans to racism and segregation, while also encouraging Blacks to improve their hygiene and living quarters and to embrace modern medicine (Summers, 2014). The National Association of Colored Women, formed in 1896 and headed by middle-class black women, was especially active in health care. They saw racial uplift as their mission, especially helping African Americans conform to mainstream social and cultural values in order to challenge racial stereotypes. They were joined by a host of other black professionals, such as social workers, midwives, club women, and educators. By 1915 a National Negro Health Week had been established.

Although the field of nursing began to flourish with the rise of hospitals and was defined as a female occupation, African-American women found it difficult to get training and employment in the field. No nursing school in the South accepted black applicants and only a few in the North did. Due to the activism of black doctors and other community leaders, Provident Hospital in Chicago was established for black students in 1891, and others followed. In 1899 the New England Hospital for Women and Children in Boston graduated six black nurses, including the first black graduate nurse in the country, Mary Eliza Mahoney (Morais, 1968). Nurses in general and black nurses in particular faced major obstacles to finding jobs after they graduated from nursing school. The hospitals that had exploited their labor as trainees had little incentive to hire them once they completed their training. Mary Carnegie, a black nurse who graduated in 1937, recalled that only about four of the 200 hospitals in the metropolitan New York City employed black nurses, and two of them assigned black nurses only to care for black patients in the tuberculosis wards (Carnegie, 1985).

Challenging segregated medicine

Although a segregated medical care system lasted until the 1960s—nearly 100 years after the abolition of slavery—African-American doctors, communities, and activist organizations worked to both challenge segregation and develop health facilities to address the immediate health care needs of the black population. With substantial funding from several foundations (for example, Rockefeller, Rosenwald, Duke Endowment), black physicians managed to establish health care facilities for black people in most communities, especially in southern and rural areas (Beardsley, 1990). Despite these efforts, the black health deficit seemed to grow in the early decades of the 20th century, much of it related to the massive northward migration of African Americans. Northward migration disrupted families and undermined health, even more so when migrants failed to find jobs and better living conditions.

The Great Depression of the 1930s led to a severe reduction of health care resources, and most African Americans who migrated North experienced a decline in health. For example, by 1940, death rates for Blacks were 33 percent higher than for Whites. Life expectancy for white males and females had risen to 62.1 and 66.6 years, compared to 51.5 for black men and 54.9 for black women. Prior to the Second World War, numerous black deaths were attributed simply to "ill-defined conditions," and as late as 1940, black deaths from "unknown causes" were ahead of cancer as a leading cause of death among African Americans (Beardsley, 1990). The economic decline facing the nation led the federal government to pass New Deal policies and the Social Security Act to spur job development and provide welfare benefits to the elderly and poor. Although some black people benefited from these policies, racial politics ensured that they did so minimally. Many Blacks were ineligible for old age assistance because they worked in farming or as domestic servants, and those who were eligible often received lower benefits based on the fact that they had a lower standard of living (Quadagno, 2000).

The entry of the US into the Second World War sparked a surge in manufacturing jobs, ended the Great Depression, and brought new opportunities for black physicians and nurses. About 1.2 million African Americans served in the War, which led the federal government to increase the number of black medical personnel. By the end of the war, about 600 black doctors and 500 black nurses had been incorporated into the armed forces. The economic standing of most Americans, including African Americans, improved after the Second World War due to a thriving industrial economy. Still, by 1949 the median black household income was still only 51 percent of that for white households (Morais, 1968).

The Second World War and the post-war economic affluence produced more opportunities for black doctors and nurses, but did not eliminate the segregated medical system. However, the National Association for the Advancement of Colored People (NAACP) won some impressive victories in the 1940s and the 1950s that opened more medical schools to African Americans. It successfully sued the University of Arkansas for refusing to admit black medical students, forcing it to integrate, and a few other states followed (Shea and Fullilove, 1985). During the 1940s, support for a national health care system that included the black population found a powerful advocate in Oscar R. Ewing, head of the Federal Security Agency. In 1940, only 9 percent of black people had hospital insurance, compared to 50 percent of white people, and the health profile of African Americans was a major factor in the nation's mortality and morbidity statistics (Thomas, 2011). Arguing that the facts of Negro health "reveal a picture of needs, misery, and desperation almost beyond belief," Ewing said:

> We have no right to be complacent about that. The life of the poorest Negro is just as important to him as yours is to you, or mine to me. His death means as much grief and sorrow to his family as your or my death would mean to our loved ones. (quoted in Thomas, 2011: 252-3)

Nevertheless, the federal government had begun to invest huge sums of money into health care, especially the construction of hospitals, but without challenging racial segregation. In 1946 the Hospital Survey and Construction Law (or the Hill-Burton Act) established hospitals and health clinics for the underserved, but it included a "separate but equal" clause that led to the creation of separate hospitals and facilities for black people. By 1974 the Hill–Burton program had distributed more than $3.7 billion to states and generated an additional $9.1 billion in local and state matching funds (Quadagno, 2000). The South received a significant share of those funds, which enabled states to actually strengthen their racially segregated facilities. The NAACP filed numerous lawsuits challenging the use of federal and state funds for racially segregated facilities, but were unsuccessful as hospitals were classified as private entities (Quadagno, 2000).

By the mid-1950s, protest against racial segregation became the focus of an organized civil rights movement that led to the Civil Rights Act in 1964. Since that time, more attention has been devoted to racial inequalities in health and the health care system. One significant study of the era, published by Harvard University Health Services in 1966, reported that serious mental and physical diseases were so common among African Americans that they seemed normal, including rat bites, rotted teeth, parasitic diseases, and developmental disorders (Morais, 1968: 154). Significant efforts were initiated to create a racially integrated medical system, including a 1965 amendment to the Hill–Burton Act ending federal funding for racially segregated hospitals. Many southern hospitals resisted the policy and developed new strategies for maintaining racially segregated facilities. However, the incentive to integrate grew when the federal government passed Medicaid and Medicare, providing millions of dollars to cover the medical expenses of the poor and elderly, but prohibiting the distribution of those funds to segregated health care facilities (Quadagno, 2000).

In 1966 all US medical schools opened to African-American students, some instituting policies of affirmative action to recruit racial minorities, and in 1968 the AMA accepted African Americans as members. Between 1971 and 1976 the Robert Wood Johnson Foundation provided $10 million to medical schools as scholarships for minorities, women, and rural medical students (Shea and Fullilove, 1985). Some of these initiatives, however, have waned in recent years, due to challenges to affirmative action policies and less funding for medical schools. Occupational segregation has also continued to be a problem, with slightly more than half of the nearly 28,000 black physicians in the US concentrated in the lower paying and less prestigious medical fields—family medicine, obstetrics-gynecology, internal medicine, and pediatrics. The income gap between black and white physicians was constant between the 1960s and the 2000s, with African-American physicians earning about 70 to 77 percent as much as white physicians, largely explained by specialty field and the racial composition of patients (Kornrich, 2009).

Conclusion

The health deficit experienced by African Americans dates at least back to slavery, which defined black people as chattel and propagated numerous theories that explained their poor health in terms of racial inferiority. This theme was given scientific merit during the early formation of the medical system and especially in the decades following the abolition of slavery. Although there has been significant progress in challenging these racial theories and dismantling the segregated medical system, the black–white racial disparity has persisted. The following part of this book looks at how it is perpetuated by health behaviors, social settings, and health policies.

Part Two
Health and medicine

Although the rise of sociology as a discipline coincided with the rise of scientific medicine, neither health nor the modern health care system were explicit topics of investigation among early sociologists. It was not until the 1930s that one of the most influential sociologists of the era, Talcott Parsons, began a series of studies that focused on illness and what he called "medical economics." He identified medicine as a vital aspect of the social structure, acknowledging that a healthy population was necessary for the effective functioning of society (Gerhardt, 1989). Parsons advanced the notion that sickness was a form of social deviance to be controlled by physicians and the medical system, whose authority and dominance he saw as appropriate. One of Parsons' earliest and most enduring contributions to the then nascent field of medical sociology was the sick role concept, which placed the study of sickness on sociological terrain by theorizing it as governed by explicit social norms and expectations. The sick role concept has since been widely critiqued on multiple bases, such as its cross-cultural relevance and applicability to chronic illnesses. Still, Parsons' work was crucial to the development of medical sociology, which, by the 1960s, had become the single most popular subfield of sociology.

This introduction to Part Two (Chapters Three and Four) of the book provides a theoretical and historical context for some key concepts and research in medical sociology. It lays the foundation for a discussion of these concepts in contemporary context, especially as they relate to the health and health care experiences of African Americans. Sociologists brought a structural perspective to the study of health and medicine by focusing on how social and economic factors influence health, but they also embraced social psychological perspectives and sometimes produced work that resonated with the culture of poverty thesis. One early example of a social structural approach to health that was pivotal in establishing the field of medical sociology was published by Faris and Dunham in the 1930s (Faris and Dunham, 1939). Using an ecological approach, they proved that patterns of mental illness in the city of Chicago varied systematically by zones, with a steady decline in insanity as one moved from the center of the city to the periphery. They argued that insanity was a result of the nature of life within the zone, especially disintegration and absence of social control, rather than the ethnicity, race, or social class of the population. During the 1990s this focus on the connection between health and neighborhoods was revived by medical sociologists, and Chapter Three examines environmental influences on health.

Medical sociologists have also focused on the more social psychological and cultural factors that affect health. During the 1940s and 1950s, most aligned themselves with the medical system and conducted research meant to solve medical problems (Gerhardt, 1989; Cockerham, 2016). By the 1950s scientific medicine, having discovered interventions to control many infectious diseases, was at the height of its popularity, and the medical community was interested in knowing why so many people did not take advantage of preventive health care services. Social scientists came to their aid and, drawing on existing research, developed the health belief model. The model originated with Irwin Rosenstock and his colleagues, who noted that their goal was to "increase the proportion of people who consistently, rationally, and freely take preventive actions or actions to check on the presence of disease while free of symptoms" (Rosenstock, 1966: 111).

The health belief model was primarily a social-psychological approach to understanding the use of preventive health services that theorized people were more likely to do so when they believed they were susceptible to contracting a serious disease. They found that people who were white, affluent and educated were more likely to access preventive care, and that those who were older, male, and less educated were least likely to do so—a finding that still holds true today. Although they realized that some people faced greater barriers to using such care, they nevertheless saw accessing preventive care as a "rational choice." Consistent with the culture of poverty thesis, they noted that lower-income people were less likely to do so because it required a future orientation, deliberate planning, and delayed gratification.

The health belief model was especially popular during the "medical era" (Cockerham, 2016), an era when having good health was largely equated with accessing medical care, especially early screening for diseases and physical exams. Today, the disease burden has shifted from infectious diseases to chronic illnesses, many of which are incurable and must be managed rather than healed. Heart disease, which has now emerged as the leading cause of death in the US, was the focus of the

Framingham Study, a longitudinal study launched in 1948 (Cockerham, 2016). Along with other research, it identified a number of factors related to the onset of heart disease, such as cigarette smoking, sedentary lifestyles, and the consumption of high fat diets. This research has been widely embraced by the health care community and the public, and the health belief model is now applied to understanding the personal and social factors that lead people to adopt better health behaviors. In this part of the book, I draw on interview data and extant research to show how African Americans define health and engage in health behaviors.

In a classic article published in the mid-1950s, Robert Strauss presciently described a division that was emerging between medical sociologists who engaged in research guided by the objectives of the medical system and those who used a sociological perspective to critique the organization of the medical system and its social processes. The former were engaged in what Strauss called sociology *in* medicine, mostly applied research addressing medical problems, while those in the sociology *of* medicine had a more theoretically driven and critical stance on the medical system (Strauss, 1957). The sociology *in* medicine perspective dominated until the 1960s, guided largely by a structural functionalist view that rarely challenged the organization or dominance of medicine. It often focused on mental illness and aligned with psychiatry. However, an anti-psychiatry movement emerged as a challenge to the medical model of mental illness. Proponents of the movement argued that in the effort to find and eradicate illnesses, medicine had created moral entrepreneurs who constructed illnesses that formerly did not exist (Freidson, 1960). Especially provocative was the work of Thomas S. Szasz, a psychiatrist who claimed that mental illness was a myth because it lacked a biological or physiological basis (Szasz, 1961). Critical theorists often argued that improvements in health and longevity were more due to better sanitation and nutrition than medical care, and emphasized the iatrogenic sicknesses that were caused by medical interventions (Illich, 1976).

These critiques reflected the growing dominance of a sociology *of* medicine perspective, and symbolic interactionism and social conflict theory became the major theories in medical sociology. Challenging the biomedical model of sickness as an objective, scientifically based reality, symbolic interactionism provided the framework for exploring the subjectivity of the illness experience, as people interpret illness symptoms in social and cultural context. In Chapter Four I draw on my research on sickle-cell disease to illustrate this subjectivity, and how racial and cultural factors influence the interpretation of illness, especially in responding to a stigmatized disease. Symbolic interactionism also highlights the political and social nature of illness, including the social construction of medical knowledge and diagnoses (Gerhardt, 1989). One illustration of this is how sickle-cell disease, although initially diagnosed in 1910, went from near invisibility to a major health crisis during the political activism of the 1960s, a topic discussed further in this section. Although this meant taking seriously a health issue that was once ignored, it also raised questions on medicalization and the expanding power of the medical system.

Social conflict theorists used a Marxist framework to criticize the profit-driven medical care system in the US, which leads to excessive costs, a duplication of services, and the maldistribution of health care resources (Waitzkin, 1983). The absence of a national health care system in the US and the notion of medical care as a commodity to be purchased rather than a right of citizens have been major issues for critical theorists. Although there were a few early efforts in the US to offer government-sponsored medical care to certain segments of the population, like military veterans, efforts to establish a broader publicly funded health insurance system always met fierce resistance, especially from the American Medical Association (AMA). In 1945, 75 percent of Americans were in favor of a national health insurance plan, but by 1949 that support had declined to 21 percent (Quadagno, 2009). Quadagno attributed the decline in support to the opposition of the AMA, but noted that organized labor, who wanted to negotiate health insurance as a fringe benefit for workers, also failed to support national health insurance. The major arguments against a state-sponsored health insurance program were that it was a move towards socialized medicine that would lead to a huge expansion of the federal budget, more government control over private industry, and a reduction in individual responsibility for health care.

During the 1960s, an era characterized by social protest over inequality, government-sponsored health programs targeting the two populations that were least likely to have health insurance were created, Medicare and Medicaid. Medicare is a federally funded program that provides health care to the elderly, regardless of their income. Medicaid is a jointly funded state and federal government program that provides health insurance for those who are low-income, and it mostly serves poor women and their children. These programs follow the logic of the nation's dual welfare system, where those who are deemed as "deserving" receive relatively generous benefits from the social insurance sector of the welfare system while the "undeserving" (the able-bodied poor) receive low, stigmatized benefits. Both Medicare and Social Security are social insurance programs thought of as entitlement programs based on employment histories. Senior citizens are eligible, regardless of their incomes. Medicaid, on the other hand, was more controversial and marginalized because it was associated with poverty and public assistance. Initially, those who received public assistance were automatically eligible for Medicaid. This changed, however, with the welfare reform policy of the mid-1990s, leaving many employed, low-income mothers ineligible for Medicaid. In Chapter Four we look at the consequences of this for low-income African Americans.

Amid a heated struggle between progressive and conservative politicians, in 2010 the US passed its first policy aimed at providing health care to all citizens, the Patient Protection and Affordable Care Act (ACA). It followed decades of debate over the spiraling cost of medical care and what do about the millions of Americans who were uninsured, despite being employed. By the 21st century, health care costs were consuming one-eighth of the nation's resources and had become the largest single business expense for many employers, who were moving towards plans that shifted more costs to employees (Quadagno, 2010). Medical care costs in the US rose from 4 percent of the gross domestic product (GDP) in 1945 to 17.6 percent in 2010, compared to about 9 percent for other economically advanced countries (Starr, 2011). The rise of the post-industrial economy also led to a curtailment of employee fringe benefits, including health care insurance. The number of firms offering health insurance to their employees fell from 66 percent in 1999 to only 60 percent in 2009 and, among small firms, only 46 percent were offering health insurance by 2009 (Quadagno, 2010).

The ACA maintained the basic elements of private insurance but set up price controls and strict guidelines about the health care services that were to be included in insurance policies. It also mandated that employers and individuals obtain health insurance, expanded eligibility for Medicaid, and set up health insurance exchanges to help low-income people pay insurance premiums. This health care reform policy was derisively dubbed "Obamacare," a name that eventually took hold among supporters and opponents. Critics have accused Obamacare of escalating the cost of health insurance and diminishing consumer choice and, more egregiously, claimed that the ACA encouraged allowing old people to die or was nothing short of a civil rights bill aimed to provide reparations for black people (Gilligan, 2015). A number of states—especially poor Southern states with conservative governors—have refused to participate in the program, despite the fact that the costs would have been subsidized by the federal government. The ACA has been the focus of numerous court challenges—to date, conservative members of Congress have advanced more than 60 initiatives to repeal the Act or have it declared unconstitutional. Slightly more than half of all Americans now support the ACA, but the racial divide in support remains stark: 50 percent of Whites and 80 percent of Blacks (Gilligan, 2015). Nevertheless, this legislation has expanded the power of the federal government to regulate the health industry and offered insurance coverage to millions of Americans.

THREE

Health behaviors in
social context

Health is defined by the World Health Organization (WHO) as a "state of complete physical, mental, and social well-being, and not merely the absence of disease or injury" (quoted in Cockerham, 2016: 10). There are more modest definitions of health, such as the ability to function, to work, or to carry out the daily activities of living, but the WHO definition resonates with the high expectations many people today have for health. Advances in medicine have contributed to better health, longer life spans, and broader definitions of what it means to be healthy. Most of the people I interviewed held these broader definitions of what it means to be healthy, and they usually linked health with having specific health behaviors. One 29-year-old mother of three described health this way:

> Health is your overall mental, physical, and emotional aspects of your life. To be healthy means to be in a good state of mind most of the time. Self-meditation or prayer is important, going to whatever higher power you believe in.

Similarly, another respondent recognized the connection between mind, body, and spirit, and offered health advice in her definition of health:

> [Health is] your lifestyle and your way of thinking. If you have a negative mindset it can stress you out or take a toll on your body. I'd advise that you eat your vegetables and try to see the best in everything. Try not to look so far ahead. Sometimes you have to take care of right now because looking too far ahead can stress people out.

Social class and education also affected how people defined health, with the less advantaged more likely to relate it more narrowly to medical care and following doctors' orders. "Good health is feeling good," said one mother, adding: "I try to do everything that the doctor tells me, like with the asthma and allergies. I try to stay out of urgent care!"

Seeking medical care and complying with medical advice was, in fact, once seen as the best way to insure good health; however, the emphasis today has shifted to adopting good health habits, especially getting exercise, eating healthier, controlling weight, and foregoing the use of tobacco. This current wave of health promotion advice began to emerge in earnest in the late 1960s, as the leading causes of sickness and death shifted from infectious diseases to chronic illnesses such as heart disease and cancer. For the most part, people, especially those who grew up in low-income families, have found the transition to healthier behaviors a challenge. As one 38-year-old mother explained:

> We didn't watch our diets at all growing up. We ate the same
> way others did—just down-home African-American food,
> but there were no limitations. I don't remember parents
> saying 'go exercise' or something like that, but today we do.

Many people grew up in families where the main goal was getting a meal on the table. Schools had gymnastic programs that promoted exercise, and children spent more time playing outside than plugged into computer games. But in recent years health behaviors are seen as requiring deliberate effort, what Peter Conrad has called the "ethos of healthicization," and much attention has been devoted to exploring who embraces healthy lifestyles, the obstacles to doing so, and linking health behaviors to health outcomes. This research makes an important contribution to understanding race- and social class-based disparities in health, but also risks decontextualizing behaviors, reinforcing the culture of poverty thesis, and blaming people for having poor health. Research has found that environmental context and social settings strongly affect the health lifestyles of individuals (Boardman et al, 2005): low-income people and African Americans are less likely to adopt the health behaviors defined by the dominant culture as optimal and, when they do, are less likely to reap the same benefits as their more affluent counterparts (Pampel et al, 2010).

This chapter examines health behaviors among African Americans, and then uses a broader perspective to place those behaviors in social context. I begin with an overview of the black health deficit, highlighting black–white racial disparities in health. I then turn to a discussion of health behaviors among my respondents, drawing on the health belief model (Rosenstock, 1966). This embodies notions of rational choice—that is, that people who believe they are suspectible to serious illnesses will adopt behaviors that will protect their health. Although proponents of the model understand that there may be obstacles to making healthy choices, William Cockerham's theory of healthy lifestyles offers a broader framework for exploring those obstacles (Cockerham, 2016). This theory explicitly looks at how life choices (health behaviors) are influenced by life chances (structural factors and social settings). In this chapter, I focus on religion and neighborhoods as two important social settings that influence health behaviors.

An overview of African–American health

Statistical data document that African Americans have a worse health profile and higher rate of death than White Americans for practically every illness. The qualitative data from the people I interviewed support this finding: of the 37 adults, only two described their health as "excellent," with most others going for "good" or "fair." Broader surveys of self-assessed health using a comparative framework have found that African Americans are nearly twice as likely as White Americans to rate their health as "fair" or "poor," and that self-rated health is a strong predictor of sickness and early death (Bratter and Gorman, 2011). Sicknesses are so common in the families of many African Americans they appear almost inevitable. As Sheryl Hadley, a 42-year-old single mother of two children, explained:

> Across the generations our health has not been good. My grandmother grew up in Arkansas and became diabetic with her first pregnancy, and has been ever since. Lots of overweight people, with diabetes and hypertension. It's a hereditary thing.

Middle-class African Americans have a better health profile than their less affluent counterparts, but many report serious health challenges as common in their families. Rosemary Brinks, for example, is a 44-year-old married mother who has two children, lives in a suburban area, and has a well-paying job. She described her own health as "good," although she suffers from a herniated disc and high blood pressure. Asked about the health of her siblings, she said: "My oldest brother had leukemia and my sister passed away in 2008 with complications from lupus. One of my sisters had breast cancer, but she is a survivor of that." These health narratives resonate with numerous studies that have found chronic illnesses and early death prevalent among African Americans.

The two leading causes of death in the US, heart disease and cancer, strike black people at an earlier age than for white people and, among Blacks, both are more likely to lead to premature death. Heart failure before the age of 50 is 20 times more common for black women than for white women (Williams, 2012). But gender matters: black men have a lower risk of cardiovascular disease than white men (Muennig and Murphy, 2011), but a higher rate of mortality from the disease. Black men have a higher incidence of cancer than white men, including a 37 percent higher chance of developing lung cancer (Xanthos et al, 2012). Black women have lower rates of breast cancer than white women, but higher rates of mortality from the disease than any other racial group—35 percent higher than for white women (Peek et al, 2008).

African Americans are especially prone to hypertension, or high blood pressure. More than 30 percent of black people over the age of 20 have hypertension, compared to about 22 percent of white people (Cockerham, 2016). This contributes to the fact that black men have a 60 percent higher risk of mortality from strokes than white men, and those between the ages of 30-39 have a 14 times greater risk of kidney failure as a result of hypertension. Many theories have been offered to explain the high rates of hypertension among African Americans, ranging from genetic factors to health habits, but it is likely that social stress and deprivation are also implicated.

Diabetes is a major cause of sickness and death, especially among African Americans. Black women are twice as likely as white women to be diagnosed with type 2 diabetes, and black men from 20 to 50 percent more likely than white men to have diabetes (Baptiste-Roberts et al, 2007). The prevalence of these health challenges was evident for most of the people I interviewed. As one young mother explained:

> My grandfather had a heart attack in his early 40s, and after that he stopped smoking, exercised, and ate better. My grandmother had a stroke in her late 40s and lived with that until she was 59 years old, when she died of lung cancer. My father was just kind of ... well, he was a drug user, drank alcohol. He died of a stroke about six years ago; he was 61 years old. So there's not a pattern of longevity in my family.

The extent to which race affects patterns of mental illness has been a topic of some debate, especially since race and social class inequalities are so interrelated for African Americans. One study reported that almost 25 percent of African Americans have been diagnosed with a mental illness and suggested that low-income, poor health, chronic stress, and racism were mostly responsible (Ward, Clark and Heidrich 2009). Others suggest that once differences in poverty and exposure to unfair treatment are accounted for, racial differences in mental health are eliminated or reversed (Schulz et al, 2000).

The prevalence of HIV/AIDS is widespread in black communities, leading some to call fighting the disease the civil rights issue of the 21st century. Between 2001 and 2005, the number of people who were diagnosed with HIV/AIDs among African Americans was higher than among all other racial-ethnic populations combined, and for every age group. Black men have the highest incidence of newly diagnosed cases of AIDS, but the actual racial disparity is greatest between black and white women (Morris et al, 2009). As of 2014, more than 200,000 African Americans had died of AIDS-related diseases and, while Blacks are less than 14 percent of the population, they account for 40 percent of the deaths (Brooks, 2014). Sexually transmitted diseases have also reached epidemic levels among black people, especially among teenagers and young adults (see Chapter Seven).

Although some research examining the health deficit experienced by African Americans over the life course finds that age has a leveling effect on racial disparities, most research supports the persistent inequality or cumulative disadvantage hypothesis, the latter arguing that racial disparities in health worsen over time. If there is a leveling of racial disparities in health over the life course, it may be due to the fact that African Americans have higher rates of death during youth and mid-life, with only the healthiest reaching old age. Blacks living in high-stress neighborhoods have a greater risk of experiencing sickness and early death than more affluent African Americans (Geronimus, 2001). For example, fewer than half of 16-year-old black males living in poor urban areas survive to reach middle age. Age-specific diseases may also be more prevalent among the black elderly. One study argued that the rate of Alzheimer's disease is as much as two to three times higher among older African Americans than their white counterparts, largely due to the prevalence of obesity and diabetes, although the disease progresses more slowly among Blacks (Barnes, 2014).

Although overall patterns of health and longevity show a significant black-white disparity, it bears noting that there is considerable intraracial diversity among African Americans. Poor health in old age is influenced by a lifetime of personal experiences and structural constraints, and those who were disadvantaged during childhood have higher rates of depression, more functional limitations, and more sickness in old age (Pavalko and Caputo, 2013). Longitudinal data show that black women between the ages of 52-81 had persistently higher levels of depression than white women, although the impact was mediated by physical health, social class, and marital status (Spence et al, 2011). In 2010, the life spans for African-American women and men (78 and 71.8, respectively) were shorter than those of their white counterparts (81.3 for women and 76.5 for men) (Cockerham, 2016).

Health behaviors and lifestyles

Bethany is a 24-year-old married mother of two children, ages six and eight, and is seeking a college degree in psychology and working part-time as a before- and after-school caregiver at a nearby school. While she was growing up, her parents had only two rules about food: you had to sit down at the table and eat together, and clean your plate before getting any dessert. Bethany's mother's side of the family has always been "about health and taking care of yourself," she said, describing them as "fish oil and vitamin people." Bethany pays attention to her own health and that of her children, especially since her eight-year-old daughter was diagnosed with attention deficit hyperactive disorder (ADHD) a few years ago. She describes health and her behaviors this way:

> [Health is] being able to exercise, eat right, get good sleep. Preventing yourself from getting colds, taking vitamins, good nourishment. I get most of the [health] information from the doctors' offices, schools, and grocery stores. I seek health information sometimes—I read labels before I buy stuff. I look at the nutritional facts and that shapes my behavior, somewhat. If it will help my health and I like it, I'd get it. I don't drink pop, nothing carbonated, and we don't have juices in the house. I always grab a piece of fruit during the day and for dinner we always have a vegetable. I don't overeat junk food and stuff. Exercise, eat well, and rest are the top things I do for good health.

Most of the people I spoke with across social classes are aware of the importance of health behaviors—not surprising in an era where the culture is saturated with information about taking care of your health through diet and exercise. Other than having had recent surgery on both knees, 62-year-old Brenda describes her own health as good, and explains what she does to maintain that health:

> I try to eat right, and watch Dr Oz. They say he's a big source of misinformation! I try to exercise and get magazines about health and stay active. I try to eat healthy, but I don't restrict my diet too much. I try not to bake a lot of sweets.

Most of those in the middle class have tried to make some changes in their diets and health lifestyles in order to improve their health and the health challenges that often accompany aging are often a catalyst to those efforts. As one 67-year-old women said:

> Only in the last ten years have I become more health conscious and eating differently than how I was raised. I sense that my body is responding better to the changes I'm making—I've cut out flour, sugar, dairy—not completely—but I have noticed a difference. My body responds better now.

The obesity epidemic

One of the most challenging aspects of embracing healthier lifestyles is weight control: some estimate that, when considering money spent on gym memberships, diet foods and drinks, and weight loss programs, Americans spend about $60 billion annually trying to lose weight. The rate of obesity has increased dramatically in recent years, with nearly one-third of all adults in the US being defined as overweight (Walker and Gordon, 2013). Obesity is related to nearly all chronic illnesses, especially diabetes and cardiovascular disease, and to some cancers (Umberson et al, 2009). It is one of the major health issues in the nation.

In 2013 the AMA defined obesity as a disease, a decision that was not without controversy given its medical and economic implications (Cockerham, 2016). The risk of obesity is not evenly distributed in the population, but strongly influenced by social class and race. Those with the lowest incomes are the most likely to be obese, and this is especially true for women. The highest rates of obesity are found among black women—nearly 55 percent are overweight, compared to 32.5 percent for white females. Much of this reflects the fact that many black women have low incomes, but their rates of obesity are higher than those of white women across income categories.

To some extent, obesity among African Americans, especially women, can be understood in a cultural context. Historically, African-American women often have equated having "big bodies" with strength and attractiveness, and for many it remains a cultural norm (Hill 2009). As one respondent said, "I wouldn't say there's a weight issue in our family, but we are all big women." Many African Americans describe people as "big boned" rather than fat, implying that certain body types are meant to carry more weight. The notion has some scientific merit: what is defined as an ideal weight may be based more on white body types and, in fact, black people do have bones that are 7-15 percent denser than those of white people (Bonilla-Silva, 2012). But "soul food" cooking traditions also matter, and they contradict dieting, or at least make it difficult. People form and solidify family bonds around meals, especially eating foods that are culturally defined as appealing. Being able to cook special dishes is a source of status:

> The only thing I can say is that when people get together they like to eat and fix rich, heavy foods—not salads or anything healthy.... On a holiday, there's one green vegetable and a ton of rich carbohydrate or starchy food, and corn pudding.... I've tossed around the idea of healthier options, but sometimes healthier options just don't get it.... And guess what? It affects you socially if you don't fix something good, because no one wants to eat it or give you compliments. We don't bond over salads.

Across class boundaries, Africans Americans eat fewer fruits and vegetables, more deep-fried foods, and more snacks that require little special preparation; however, poverty and living in segregated neighborhoods contribute to those food choices and obesity (Bahr, 2007). These environments have been described as obesogenic, as they promote the overconsumption of unhealthy foods and offer fewer opportunities for physical activity (Lim and Harris, 2015). These eating patterns are passed on to children, whose rates of obesity have tripled in the past three decades. Childhood obesity is related to poverty, welfare receipt, poor sleeping patterns, and parents' educational level, as well as the inability of parents to monitor their children's food choices (Lee et al, 2009).

Despite these obstacles, studies find that nearly 70 percent of obese African-American women are attempting to lose weight, although weight loss intervention programs have rarely been successful (Walker and Gordon, 2013). Almost all of the women I spoke with felt they should lose weight but, like most Americans, they struggled with adopting the health behaviors that would help them do so:

> I am overweight. I should be walking right now, but I'm here with you…. Over the years I have continued to gain weight due to lack of exercise and eating [habits] … at times I've lost 30-something pounds, but then an issue might happen … and I'm motivated to eat up. A great many women in my family are overweight. I'm an emotional eater.

The struggle becomes even more intense and stressful when people are diagnosed with illnesses that are directly related to obesity. Asked to describe her health, 46-year-old Mason said:

> My health is below average; I have some issues. I have diabetes, which is under control right now. I have had it for 10 or 15 years. And I have high blood pressure. I had gastric bypass and lost 87 pounds, so that put everything under control. But now I've gained 25 pounds—I got pregnant right after having the bypass, so I wasn't able to get down to my ideal weight. So I am still about 75 pounds over. I am flunking on healthy eating, because I'm a stress eater. Work is stressful—I don't especially like what I'm doing, but it's a job—then coming home to take care of my family—I'm overwhelmed. It just makes me want to eat, eat, eat, though I know I'm not hungry. Right now I'm trying to fast on a liquid high protein diet, I want to do it for two weeks.

Mason has a good paying job but it requires her to be at work at 3.45 in the morning and to stay until the job is done, which typically means two to three hours of overtime each day. The job is stressful, and it interferes with her ability to care for her two children.

Health behaviors in social context

In 2005 Hurricane Katrina struck the Gulf Coast of the US causing massive destruction and loss of life. Nearly 700 people died as a result of the hurricane—most of them African Americans—and about 75 percent of those who were reported missing were Black. Hurricane Katrina became the topic of much political debate and scholarly research, as it represented a dismal government response to a disaster that overwhelmingly affected poor and black people. But while some decried the avoidable loss of life, others blamed residents for failing to evacuate when ordered to do so. Using the health belief model as a framework, one study used focus groups to examine why low-income black men living in New Orleans failed to evacuate (Elder et al, 2007). The results revealed that many believed they could ride the storm out because of earlier experiences with hurricanes or because of their religious faith. But they also named a number of cultural and structural factors that influenced their decisions, such as the timeliness of the evacuation order, the fear that police officers would not protect their property, and the lack of resources (for example, money and gas) required to leave.

The study reveals some of the limitations of the health belief model, which assumes that people would have behaved to the threat of death by fleeing. Instead, while people do have choices, they are often constrained by life chances. William Cockerham's theory of health lifestyles uses both to explore why people may or may not engage in health behaviors. Life choices (human agency), he has pointed out, intersect with life chances (social and structural forces), which are shaped by many factors, most saliently structural inequalities in economic resources, schools, living conditions, and neighborhoods. Racial minorities and lower-income people often did not grow up with nor do they have the same life chances as those who are more economically advantaged, and this influences their health behaviors. People across class and racial lines have some awareness of what they should do to take care of their health, but the more educated and affluent tend to be more knowledgeable about health issues and face fewer barriers to implementing that knowledge.

Social class, especially as measured by education, is the most important variable in shaping health attitudes and behaviors: lower-income and less educated people engage in fewer positive health behaviors than those who are educated and affluent, often because they face more obstacles in doing. One is varying levels of health literacy, defined as the ability to obtain and understand basic health information and services. African Americans as a group score lower on health literacy than Whites (Rowland and Isaac-Savage, 2014), even those who are college-educated (Bennefield, 2015). In some cases, such as seeking treatment for mental illness, they underutilize health services unless they learned about mental illness by having a family member diagnosed with it (Villatoro and Aneshensel, 2014).

This lack of knowledge about health issues is also heightened by the fear of discovering an illness. Asked "what keeps you from doing what you should to stay healthy?" a focus group composed of African-American men living in a low-income neighborhood in Chicago noted a lack of health awareness of disease signs and symptoms. But they also feared medical procedures and receiving adverse diagnoses: "Knowing things adds to your problems," one man explained: "The more you know, the more you have to think about. As long as I'm healthy, I don't want to think about it" (quoted in Ravenell et al, 2008).

More than health knowledge, however, are structural inequalities that perpetuate differences in health and health behaviors. Poor people and African Americans across the social class spectrum have more stressful living and working conditions, which promotes risky health behaviors. Delores Jones grew up in a middle-class family with two parents who "smoked like chimneys" and both died early of massive heart attacks. Her sister continues to smoke, exposing the granddaughter who lives with her and has asthma to secondhand smoke and jeopardizing her own health. Delores explains:

> My sister is a very nervous person, and I guess that's her coping. I noticed this weekend she had an electric cigarette of some kind.... I said [to her] 'Do you realize how blessed you are, all your Creator has brought you through?'—a mastectomy, then she had quadruple bypass surgery, and then she had this surgery to open the veins of her legs because her toes were so dark—and her fingers, you know, were not getting enough oxygen.

Delores attributes her sister's behavior to coping with nervousness and stress, often the result of powerlessness and marginalization. Stress and experiencing adverse events make giving up risky health behaviors difficult: even when they are costly (for example, buying cigarettes), they are seen as coping or mood controlling (Pampel et al, 2010).

Income and education are most often used as measures of social class, but social class groups are also status groups, where prestige is determined by specific patterns of consumption, lifestyles, and cultural behaviors. Based on structural location class-status groups develop their own norms about issues such as smoking, exercising, and eating, and some behaviors that are more stigmatized among those who are middle-class (for example, smoking cigarettes, being overweight) are more acceptable among the less privileged. More affluent people gain more from engaging in healthy lifestyles than the poor—longer lives, better careers, and more financial advantages (Pampel et al, 2010). These scholars found that health behaviors are important but ultimately account for only about 25 percent of the class-based gap in health.

Still, the seemingly volitional nature of these behaviors pave the way for blaming the poor for having poor health, especially in the context where good health is seen as an individual achievement. The ethos of individual responsibility reinforces the ideological shift from welfare liberalism to neoliberalism, which emphasizes reduced public support for human welfare services and more personal responsibility for health. It also protects existing power relations by ignoring entrenched social class and racial inequalities and the social conditions that perpetuate them (Baum and Fisher, 2014). Research, however, consistently finds that health lifestyles do not exist in a vacuum, but are linked to social environments and settings (Boardman et al, 2005; Frohlich and Abel, 2014).

Religion and health

Cockerham has pointed out that health attitudes and behaviors are shaped by social factors as well as collectivities, or "thought communities," that link people together based on shared beliefs. Religion constitutes one such community, and studies across the decades have shown that there is a positive relationship between good health and religiosity. In the early 1900s one of the founders of scientific medicine, Sir Willian Osler, wrote of the healing power of faith, a belief embraced by all major religions (Levin, 2009). Most scholars have been more circumspect on the question of direct intervention from God in answering prayers, but have found a number of reasons why religion promotes good health and longevity. One of the more obvious is that people involved in religion tend to embrace better health behaviors; for example, they are less likely to smoke tobacco or use drugs or alcohol.

Religion also promotes hope, optimism, and positivity—attitudes and dispositions that decrease social stress and build confidence. A study by David H. Rosmarin found that among psychiatric patients the belief in God, regardless of religious affiliation, resulted in lower levels of depression and self-harm and higher levels of psychological wellbeing (Rosmarin et al, 2013). Amy M. Burdette examined how attending religious services affected one of the most important problems facing black, low-income mothers—adverse birth outcomes. She found that, regardless of their health behaviors, those who attended religious services regularly were less likely to have low birth weight infants, a favorable result that has health benefits across generations (Burdette et al, 2012).

African Americans have long been known to have high levels of religiosity and religious participation (Holt and McClure, 2006). Data for 2015 from the Pew Institute found that 53 percent of Americans say religion is very important in their lives, with Blacks (75 percent) more likely than Whites (49 percent) to express that sentiment. Most people who are religious believe that God—or a Supreme Being—directly intervenes in their lives, bringing health, healing, and other blessings. I have met very few people (other than Christian Scientists) who have given up on the medical system in favor of relying solely on prayer for healing, but there are some. One respondent told me that her mother, then in her early 60s, was diagnosed with ovarian cancer five years ago; declining medical treatment, she "claimed her healing" by faith in God and has experienced no decline in her health.

Black churches are places not only for creating community and sharing spiritual beliefs, but also where being connected to a religious community often improves health through social affiliations and support. Members accumulate religious social capital that comes from being part of a network, a cohesive community with a shared set of interests and values (Maselko et al, 2011).

The black church has long been a place not only for sharing spiritual beliefs, but also where black cultural traditions are maintained and racial solidarity is reinforced. Many were rallying points for the civil rights movement, and they continue to engage in social justice work, thus fostering a sense of empowerment. Traditional black churches often have open testimony services, where emotional venting is common. Worship styles encourage high levels of participation and spontaneity, including dancing, interacting, singing, and speaking in tongues, all of which are conducive to good health (Musick et al, 2004). For many black people, church membership and service provides a source of status and esteem that is often unavailable in other arenas of life. In church they garner respect by holding responsible, highly visible roles as church leaders, teachers, and pastors (Musick, House, and Williams 2004).

Embracing religious teachings can serve as a coping strategy for dealing with the difficulties of life, especially persistent health challenges and sicknesses. They allow people to cope with incurable health issues and redefine the meaning of health. As one person with multiple sclerosis interviewed by Holt and McClure explained:

> But [God] still had a plan for everybody's life and though we are healthy even though we may get an illness we can still be spiritually healthy.... Even if you're in a wheelchair with multiple sclerosis you can still be a positive force ... showing the world that I have MS, but I'm still healthy. (quoted in Holt and McClure, 2006: 268)

Religious institutions also directly address questions of health through sermons and health promotion campaigns. Studies find that the content of sermons in black churches frequently link spirituality and health, as pastors share stories from their own experiences in pursuing good health and allow the use of the church for health care activities (Barnes, 2013; Lumpkins et al, 2014). Rowland and Isaac-Savage (2014) surveyed 100 black churches and found that the majority of them offered health care materials that specifically pertained to African Americans, and most had some type of health and screening program. The use of churches for health promotion activities, in fact, has been supported by federal government-sponsored faith-based and neighborhood partnership funds aimed at merging religion and disease prevention activities.

Beyond providing health initiatives, most churches offer tangible support for their members through support groups and financial aid. Elderly Blacks, especially women, have a higher rate of church affiliation than any other racial group, and the majority of them receive direct assistance from their churches, ranging from financial help to emotional support and advice (Chatters et al, 2014). Thus, there is an extensive literature that supports the health benefits of religiosity, faith, and active involvement in religious communities, and it documents the use of religious settings to promote good health behaviors. It bears noting, however, that religious ideologies and institutions may also lead to beliefs and behaviors that are antithetical to good health. Many people, for example, believe that sickness can be the result of insufficient faith or sin, leading to guilt and self-blame. Religions that lean towards conservativism often embrace patriarchal and gender traditions that are out of step with contemporary society; for example, they teach male headship of families, endorse subordinate roles for women, and believe that only men should hold key leaderships roles in the church, such as pastor, elder, or deacon.

Traditional churches often reject progressive attitudes about reproductive rights, the use of birth control, and abortion rights. Non-marital sex, although now a cultural norm, is seen as sinful regardless of the age or consent of participants, and the promotion of chastity (especially for single females) precludes frank discussions about sex or the epidemic of sexually transmitted diseases that plague young African Americans. Many churches also condemn and marginalize people who are homosexual or involved in same-sex relationships, denying them acceptance, respect, and the right to hold certain positions in the church, such as choir member or teacher. The discovery of HIV/AIDS, which was initially narrowly linked to same-sex behavior among gay men, has led to more stigma and condemnation. One study of clergy responses to those with HIV/AIDS found that people who have the disease are shunned in some congregations, as one pastor explained:

> Individuals don't wanna sit by 'em on the pew, don't want to eat anything they bring to the church. They frown when they are in their presence. They embrace them lightly instead of with a good—full embrace or hug. That's a stigma to us. (quoted in Aholou et al, 2016)

Pastors often said they were unaware of congregants or others who had HIV/AIDS until it was too late to reach out to them.

Neighborhoods and health

Living conditions, especially the neighborhood in which one lives, have a major impact on health. Neighborhoods vary significantly in terms of the quality of schools, the availability of resources (for example, employment, health care, transportation, play areas for children), levels of safety, and social relationships between residents. Racial segregation in housing has been the historic norm in the US, and African Americans generally have been restricted to housing in the poorest and often most deprived neighborhoods. Nevertheless, many African Americans remember the neighborhoods of the 1950s and 1960s as safe areas where residents knew and trusted each other, and collectively asserted social control over the activities of children. Accounts like that given by Josie Avalon, who grew up in the 1950s, were common:

> Oh, it [the neighborhood] was great ... it was a community, you knew everybody in your block, you knew families, you played with their kids. I lived across the stress from the park, and sometimes I would sneak out to other neighborhoods, to get to their fruit trees, and people would call my dad ... and tell him I wasn't supposed to be there, and that's the way it was. If you were someplace you weren't supposed to be, they would call your parents.... My dad and I would walk down to the movies and then walk back. You could be out at night and people didn't worry ... there was no fear.

The emphasis on solidarity, trust, and safety explain the nostalgia many people express over the communities they grew up in, and that sentiment is also found among people who grew up in white ethnic communities. Many of these neighborhoods, especially those occupied by Blacks, had substandard and overcrowded houses and poor access to city services. But for those moving from the rural South—where living in shacks and former slave cabins was common—it was an improvement in their standard of living. Many came from areas without running water, electricity, and indoor toilets, so access to urban amenities was a step upward. But what people remember the most was knowing and watching out for each other, creating an environment that was relatively safe for children. These neighborhoods had collective efficacy or intergenerational closure, defined as "social ties between parents of interconnected youth, attachment to community, and norms regulating adolescent behavior" (Browning et al, 2008: 270).

The flood of African Americans moving into urban areas helped spark suburbanization, most of which took place after the Second World War and was heavily subsidized by federal government. But with racial segregation in housing (and the rest of society) still the norm, few black people benefited from the expanded housing market. Realtors practiced redlining (the practice of denying services, either directly or through selectively raising prices, to residents of certain areas based on the racial or ethnic makeups of those areas), and honored racially restrictive housing policies that channeled African Americans to poor and deteriorating neighborhoods. An influential book by Oliver and Shapiro attributed racial gaps in wealth and homeownership largely to the explicit policies of the federal government, which embraced these practices (Oliver and Shapiro, 1995). The federal government implemented New Deal policies in the 1930s to refinance tens of thousands of homes that were on the very brink of default due to the Great Depression. It later created the Federal Housing Authority

(FHA), which made low-interest, no money down loans to prospective homeowners. But the policies were confined to suburban areas, the significant majority of which were all-white neighborhoods.

Policy-makers contended that in order to achieve stability, neighborhoods had to be occupied by the same social and racial classes (Oliver and Shapiro, 1995). Of the more than $120 billion in new housing financed by the FHA between 1934 and 1962, only 2 percent went to non-Whites. The passage of the Fair Housing Act in 1968, which forbade housing discrimination, resulted in a decline in racial segregated housing, but the decline has been smallest in those areas where black people are most likely to live. Although many of those in the middle class have left the poorest and most racially segregated sections of the city, African Americans continue to be more geographically segregated from Whites than other racial groups (Burton et al, 2010).

Neighborhood influences on health

The relationship between health and neighborhood quality has been recognized at least since the public health campaigns of the early 1900s, but research on the issue re-emerged in the 1970s. Middle-class Blacks increasingly left urban neighborhoods, leaving behind their poorer counterparts. The social bonds and sense of community that once existed in black neighborhoods diminished, and inner-city areas increasingly became known for housing the so-called "underclass"— single mothers who were dependent on public assistance and young black men who, disconnected from the labor market, were increasingly involved in crime, violence, and drug use. Homicide rates in black neighborhoods soared during the 1970s and 1980s, and they have remained high. In 2011, the overall rate of black homicide victimization was 17.51 per 100,000, compared to 4.4 for all Americans and 2.64 for White Americans. Gun violence accounted for 82 percent of the homicides (Sugarmann, 2014).

The concept of neighborhood disadvantage has been widely used in research exploring racial and class disparities in health. The premise is that certain neighborhood characteristics, such as social disorder, can affect health. Catherine Ross maintained that neighborhoods can be evaluated on a continuum ranging from orderly (for example, clean, safe, well-maintained, quiet, and respectful neighbors) to disorderly (noisy, littered, poorly maintained, and composed of single-parent families). Using this scale, Ross found that living in a disorderly neighborhood is strongly associated with feeling run-down, hopeless, sad, and having chronic health problems. Many people living in disadvantaged neighborhoods experience a sense of normlessness—a gap between their goals and their ability to achieve them—and more social isolation. Ross concluded that neighborhood conditions such as graffiti, noise, vandalism, vacant buildings, and dirty streets, convey messages of a lack of social worth to residents (Ross, 2000; Ross and Mirowsky, 2009).

Disadvantaged neighborhoods typically have high rates of poverty, unemployment, and single mothers relying on welfare assistance. Low rates of homeownership and marginal schools are common (Hill et al, 2005). In many poor areas, police surveillance is common, and black men are often subjected to stop-and-frisk policies. These policing policies cause high levels of psychological distress among men, leading to feelings of worthlessness and nervousness (Sewell et al, 2016). Living in a state of chronic stress explains the link between neighborhood disadvantage and poor health, according to Hill and associates (2005). Neighborhoods characterized by poverty, crime, decay, and disorder literally gets under the skin, elevating psychological and physiological stress. Exposure to chronic stress, they argued, not only leads to depression, lethargy, and hopelessness, but it also degrades physiological systems. It results in greater susceptibility to pathogens and decreases the effectiveness of the immune system and resistance to infections, leading to serious illnesses, including cancer. A study by Emily Walton found that neighborhood segregation predicts higher rates of infant mortality and low weight birth among African Americans (Walton, 2009).

Matthew Desmond has recently focused on one of the key factors related to adverse health among people living in poor neighborhoods— constantly relocating, often due to being evicted. Data show that at the national level poor people spend more than half of their income on rent, and 25 percent spend 70 percent of their income on rent (Desmond, 2016). Owning property in poor, dilipidated areas of the city has become big business, because landowners can extract exhorbitant rents from people who are desperately poor and have no place else to go. Moreover, since the renters who are poor end up owing a large portion of their income to landlords, they are likely to fall behind in their rent and thus have no leverage in forcing landlords to maintain the property. Desmond found that among renters in the city of Milwaukee, where he conducted his study, half encountered housing problems such as rodents, the lack of heat, or inadequate plumbing, with African Americans more likely to be affected. Millions are evicted every year, often in humiliating ways, such as having their front doors removed.

Living in poor and segregated neighborhoods encourages the practice of unhealthy and high-risk behaviors. Liquor stores are often concentrated in such neighborhoods, as are advertisements that promote cigarette smoking and vendors who sell cigarettes by the pack or singly. Many of these neighborhoods are saturated with fast food restaurants and convenience stores offering quick, ready-prepared food options, but are literally food deserts when it comes to finding grocers and stores offering nutritious, affordable food (Walker and Gordon, 2013). Even when grocers are available, food insufficiency is common in low-income, single-mother families. Since the welfare reform policy of 1996, the number of low-income families receiving food stamps has fallen from 27.5 million in 1994 to 17.4 million at the end of 1999; however, food insufficiency has declined by only 16 percent (Siefert et al, 2004).

Low-income black women living in Detroit lamented the decline of living standards in their neighborhood, including things like the loss of jobs and grocers in their communities and the decline in safety (Schulz and Lempert, 2004). They were well aware of what people "should do" to take care of their health—eat less fried food, exercise— but their neighborhoods were not conducive to those activities. One elderly respondent, for example, spoke of having to travel several miles by bus to get decent food, and all of them spoke of the "closed door policies" in their neighborhoods, since neighbors no longer trusted each other. Research has linked neighborhood quality to a variety of health risks, such as obesity and the early onset of sexuality (from early to middle teenage years). For example, Boardman and his associates (2005) found that in poor black neighborhoods, there is often a collective minimization of the health risks of obesity.

The exposure to health risks in poor neighborhoods is exacerbated by environmental racism and public policies that endanger the health of people in poor communities. Low-income and racial minority neighborhoods are targeted as dumping grounds for waste and environmental toxins, contributing to hazardous living conditions. The environmental justice movement originated in the 1960s as part of the civil rights movement, after an eight-year-old black girl drowned in a garbage dump in a residential area of Houston (Cole and Foster, 2001). Leaders of the movement have documented a nationwide pattern of locating waste facilities in poor and predominantly black communities, often with the promise that they would generate jobs. Cole and Foster, for example, found that between 1986 and 1996, the

Pennsylvania Department of Environmental Protection issued seven permits for commercial waste facilities, and located six of them in one poor black county. Such activities elevate feelings of social disorder and powerlessness among residents and are associated with more psychological distress and depression (Downey and van Willigen, 2005).

The disregard for the lives and health of the poor and racial minorities by many lawmakers was again evident in 2016 with the discovery that the state of Michigan had switched the water supply for people living in the predominantly poor and African-American city of Flint. To reduce the budget, state authorities decided to switch the water supply from the Huron to the Flint River, and to further save money by not treating the water with an anticorrosion agent that would have cost $100 a day, but made the water fit for consumption. Residents complained of water that looked, smelled, and tasted foul, but were assured that the water was safe. Yet over the course of two years, hundreds of people were made sick by the water, and literally thousands of children were exposed to irreversible lead poisoning—a situation many have noted could never have happened in a "wealthier, whiter" city. Physicians found that the lead blood levels in toddlers had doubled and even tripled since the change in the water supply, and documented a surge in other sicknesses. Further research has found that the residents of Flint were, in fact, exposed to a host of toxic substances in the water, leading the federal government to declare a national emergency requiring at least $1.5 billion to repair. These repairs, however, can scarcely compensate parents for the damage inflicted on their children or the loss of value in their homes caused by the crisis.

Homeownership: the American Dream

Racial segregation in housing has declined in recent years but remains greater for African Americans than any other racial groups. Although high-income African Americans are more likely now than in the past to live in integrated neighborhoods, persistent segregation is explained more by racial than class differences (Farley, 2005). Farley found that the majority of Whites prefer to live in either predominantly or all-white areas, and black people prefer to live in integrated neighborhoods. In their search for such neighborhoods, however, African Americans have fewer resources to invest in housing, and even those who are middle class often end up in neighborhoods that are only marginally better than the ones they left or are undergoing a process of decline (Pattillo-McCoy, 1999). Thus, they experience a "segregation tax" as the homes they purchase appreciate more slowly or in some cases depreciate in value (Oliver and Shapiro, 2001).

Home ownership is the major form of wealth for most Americans, and owning one's own home has always been part of the American Dream. During the 1980s and 1990s a proliferation of subprime loans for houses enabled many African Americans to become homeowners, often with disastrous results. Research has shown that through a process of reverse redlining, lenders capitalized on racial segregation by targeting African Americans for high-risk loans that were based on equity (or assets) rather than ability to pay (Oliver and Shapiro, 2008; Rugh et al, 2015). Racial discrimination shaped every stage of the lending process, from excessive startup costs and interest rates to high mortgage payments and the ultimate foreclosure on and repossession of the property (Rugh et al, 2015). In the process, African-American families faced the stress and shame of losing their homes and a significant loss of wealth, much of it lost as they struggled to hold on to the property. This represented a significant loss of wealth and the intergenerational transfer of disadvantage, with more affluent African Americans actually losing more than their low-income counterparts.

More recently scholars have implicated racially segregated housing in the persistent wealth gap that exists between Blacks and Whites. Recent data show that the typical white household has $111,146 in wealth, compared to $7,113 for the typical black household (Fletcher, 2015). In 2014, 72.3 percent of Whites lived in their own homes, compared to only 42.1 percent of Blacks. Home ownership is an especially crucial component of wealth; in fact, it accounts for about 63 percent of the wealth of black people and 38.5 percent of white wealth, as Whites are also more likely more likely than Blacks to have wealth in stocks, bonds, and other assets (Oliver and Shapiro, 2008).

Conclusion

Health promotion activities these days often focus on the need to prevent or manage illness by engaging in specific health behaviors. Medical wisdom and nutritional guidelines about what one should eat or do to promote health shift over time, but there is general constancy in beliefs such as the value of exercising, controlling weight, and foregoing cigarette smoking. These health behaviors are often the focus of health promotion activities, and there is evidence that they can improve health and lower rates of mortality. One study, for example, targeted an African-American community whose residents had a 40 percent higher rate of death from cardiovascular disease than the rest of the county, and were three times more likely to be hospitalized for diabetes. By engaging residents in the community in the project, they were able to significantly decrease cigarette smoking in the community and increase the consumption of fruits and vegetables (Plescia et al, 2008).

There is no doubt that many chronic diseases can be prevented by embracing healthier behaviors, leading Michael Marmot to claim that medicine is "failed prevention." This chapter has documented the changing health behaviors among black people and social institutions that support those changes, such as churches. On the other hand, Marmot called diseases "social disadvantage in action," pointing to the futility of treating diseases and then sending people back to the conditions that made them sick (Marmot, 2015). Nutritious diets, exercise, and other healthy behaviors may help people avoid serious illnesses, but they cannot ameliorate the adverse health consequences of unequal social and living conditions and racially biased policies that undermine the health of black people. The emphasis on health behaviors may obscure the social conditions that cause sickness and lead to more victim-blaming. The US has higher levels of health inequality than most rich countries, due mostly to notable disparities in living conditions and life chances (Halfon, 2012). This chapter has focused on health behaviors, but also the social context that fosters health and sickness. These social contexts mediate health behaviors and the extent to which such behaviors can improve health.

FOUR

Medical care and health policy

During the late 1960s Doris Jacobs was screened for sickle-cell anemia, one of several sickle-cell diseases (SCD) that primarily affect African Americans, and diagnosed with having the sickle-cell trait. The 1970s was an era when advances in medical screening technologies and political activism among African Americans merged to define sickle-cell anemia as a major epidemic among African Americans, and one that had been neglected by the health care system arguably because it was a "black disease." Indeed, sickle-cell anemia was first diagnosed in 1910, but awareness of it among health authorities or black people was uncommon. It is now known to be one of a related group of SCDs that are genetically transmitted, incurable, and, until recent decades, thought to lead to early death. The red blood cells of people with sickle-cell anemia take the shape of a sickle and become sticky, which restricts the flow of blood through the vessels. In some cases this leads to death, but the more common outcomes are relentless pain (or "pain crises"), bacterial infections, organ damage, and strokes. SCDs are now known to be the most common genetic blood disorders in the world and, in the US, affect as many as 98,000 people, mostly African Americans. About 1 in every 350 African Americans is born with the disease every year (Ciribassi and Patil, 2016).

The US SCD experience provides an interesting lens for looking at the politics of medicine and the repercussions of those politics, and how racial and class inequalities influence responses to illness symptoms and diagnoses. The SCD crisis represented another chapter in a long history of experiences that have distanced African Americans from the medical system and caused many to distrust physicians. The public and medical response to SCD, which by the late 1960s was being called a neglected epidemic among African Americans, highlighted the intersection between medicine and politics. The National Sickle Cell Anemia Control Act of 1972, passed during an era of social protest against racial segregation and injustice, described the disease as a "deadly and tragic burden" and provided the basis for a national program to screen for and treat sickle cell anemia. But with racial policies historically used to disadvantage African Americans, the Act generated a host of ethical questions: should screening for the disease be voluntary or involuntary? Would being diagnosed with SCD lead to improved access to medical care for African Americans, or more racial stigma? How would the reproductive rights of African-American women be affected if they (or their partners) were diagnosed as having SCD, or as carriers of the trait?

This chapter examines how race and racism shape illness behaviors, or the interpretation of illness symptoms and pursuit of medical care. The discussion is informed by data from my earlier study of how SCD became a major medical care issue (Hill, 1994) and the more recent interviews I conducted for this book. This chapter also focuses on the experiences of African Americans in the health care system, especially how medical mistrust and physician–patient interactions affect the use and quality of health care. These racial experiences intersect with economic factors to shape responses to sickness. Financial barriers continue to pose a significant problem for many, even those who are employed, as employment-based health insurance has become less common. Slightly more than half of employers provide health insurance as a worker benefit, and even then many of the costs of medical care are shifted back to patients. Neoliberal policies have also led to cuts in Medicaid, thus undermining access to medical care by the poor. Given these factors, it is not surprising that unpaid medical bills are the leading cause of bankruptcies in the US (Fontenot, 2014).

Interpreting symptoms of illness

Illness behaviors, as defined by David Mechanic, are the ways in which people define, interpret, and respond to either internal states or physical symptoms (Mechanic, 1995). Unlike disease, which is a biological condition, illness is much more subjective, experiential, and embedded with cultural meaning (Conrad and Barker, 2010). When people experience symptoms of illness, they engage in a process of interpreting those symptoms and deciding how to respond to them. Many people ignore or dismiss early symptoms of illness as trivial or meaningless; if the symptoms persist, they engage in some form of self-care, such as rest or over-the-counter medications. Before seeking medical care it is also common for people to use a process of lay consultation with family members or friends, who jointly construct the meaning of the symptoms based on race, class, and cultural factors (Freidson, 1960). One early study found that people who are part of closed, exclusive social networks, especially in low-income neighborhoods, are especially likely to consult among themselves in defining illness and often shun or distrust medicine (Suchman, 1965).

More recent research has also shown the importance of social networks and relationships in responding to symptoms of illness (Pescosolido, 1992). For example, social relationships have been found to be important in the diagnosis of hypertension and the effective management of the disease. People who received emotional support from family members and friends and were married were less likely to have undiagnosed hypertension (Cornwell and Waite, 2012). Health literacy also matters and varies by race and social class (Bennefield, 2015). These factors shaped the experiences of those who experienced symptoms of SCD or had children with those symptoms. Many had never heard of the disease, nor had their family members. Moreover, low-income people are simply more tolerant of illness symptoms because they are so common among those in their families and communities (Koos, 1954). African Americans have often held physically demanding jobs where aches and pains—the major symptoms of SCD—were an accepted part of life. Those in their social networks helped them normalize even persistent symptoms of illness, which were often explained and treated outside the context of the medical system. As late as the 1970s, low-income and poor Blacks were more likely to draw on a variety of folk healers than their White counterparts (Roebuck and Quan, 1976).

Race-ethnic factors also matter in the interpretation of illness symptoms and how people respond to those symptoms (Zola, 1966). African-American responses to SCD were shaped by the deeply entrenched racial policies based on the "separate but equal" doctrine, which meant African Americans often received inferior care in overcrowded, substandard facilities, or were turned away by facilities that had filled their allotted share of "black beds." These policies, along with fear of the treatment they often received at the hands of physicians, distanced many from the medical system. Having a racially specific disease in a society that already held theories of racial inferiority was another barrier to seeking care. Although many African Americans were unaware of SCD prior to the civil rights era, those who knew about it or were diagnosed with the disease often felt stigmatized.

Researchers have found that this often leads people to deny they have the disease or refuse medical care (Conrad and Barker, 2010). Denial, in fact, was seen as one of the major barriers to identifying and treating people with SCD. Some African Americans understood the disease as having "bad blood," which resonated with theories of racial inferiority. The diagnosis of sickle-cell anemia in a child—which is only possible when both parents have either the trait or the disease—disrupted families and especially led fathers to deny paternity.

Nevertheless, screening for SCD became widespread during this era. In most cases screening was brought to the African-American community through schools and churches and, especially for men, through the military and prisons. Women were also likely to be screened for SCD when they sought health care services for birth control or pregnancy, often without their consent. When a person was diagnosed with SCD, no real treatment regimen was given, other than knowing that persistent bodily pains could be serious and require medical treatment. Most people, however, were diagnosed with the trait and not expected to experience any symptoms. Thus when Doris, introduced earlier in this chapter, was told she had the sickle-cell trait, she really did not think much about the reproductive implications.

Seeking medical care

Studies of illness behaviors ultimately seek to understand pathways to seeking medical care. David Mechanic outlined several factors that usually lead people to seek medical care, such as the persistence, frequency, salience, and perceived seriousness of symptoms. When illness symptoms disrupt the daily activities of the ill person, they are more likely to lead them to seek medical care. Doris' story illustrates this. Two years after she was diagnosed with the sickle-cell trait, she had graduated from high school and had her first child. It was not until her daughter's symptoms became persistent and severe that she was diagnosed with SCD. As Doris said, "[My daughter] would cry a lot, and she'd have a lot of fevers, a lot of high fevers. And if you touched her, she didn't like it." After numerous trips to the doctor, her daughter was finally diagnosed with SCD. Although it took some persistence before the doctors discovered the problem was SCD, in the past such diagnoses were often not made until adulthood, if at all. Children who were taken to the doctor repeatedly for bodily pains received an array of explanations from medical professions, such as growing pains and poor posture. One woman who was not diagnosed with sickle-cell anemia until her teenage years said the doctor often had her sit in straight back chairs in the hospital corridor for hours to correct her posture. Adults experiencing pain crises were misdiagnosed as having severe arthritis, or suspected of exaggerating their pain in order to obtain drugs.

Understanding pathways to medical care has always been a topic of interest among medical sociologists. In 1978 Diana Dutton published a study that explored the low use of medical care among a poor, predominantly black population by testing three hypotheses: the culture of poverty thesis, the impact of financial barriers, and the impact of systems barriers. She found some support for the culture of poverty thesis, although it has been a much debated topic in the social sciences (Dutton, 1978). Many poor people do exhibit the behaviors it outlines, for example, low rates of marriage, high rates of non-marital childbearing, and a present-moment rather than future orientation. Low-income people are more likely to engage in risky health behaviors such as smoking tobacco and less likely to utilize preventive care than their middle-class counterparts. Structural factors, however, such as lack of opportunity and resources and stressful living conditions, account for these adaptive behaviors. As Ann Swidler has more recently pointed out, it is erroneous to describe the behaviors of poor people as an expression of their cultural values. Rather, most can be understood as the behaviors one draws from a toolkit for survival when society has offered them fewer opportunities (Swidler, 1986). The culture of poverty thesis is a victim-blaming framework when disconnected from its structural basis, as it fails to explore the underlying factors that produce the culture. But in addition to recognizing that the culture of poverty does shape the utilization of health care services, Dutton argued that financial barriers were much more important than cultural behaviors and systems barriers—the overall organization of health care services was the single most important factor.

Health insurance

Health care decisions are influenced by whether one has access to health insurance. When Josie Avalon found herself pregnant with her first child in the early 1960s, neither she nor her husband were covered by insurance. Her husband had just resigned from a job that did offer insurance in order to go to dental school, and Josie was not insured on her job. One can never anticipate the occurrence of an event that will require medical care, and for Josie, that event was pregnancy. After several years of marriage and fertility treatment, they had given up on having a baby, and were shocked (but happily so) when Josie became pregnant. But when she learned, late in her pregnancy, that it would be a breech birth, they both realized that they could not pay for a surgical birth. As Josie explained:

> I had a breech birth, so that wasn't good. They didn't do sonograms much—the doctor would just put his finger up there and figure out what was going on—so they didn't know. And it was hard to estimate when the baby would come, so he when decided the baby was 'butt first,' it was late in the pregnancy. So I asked if I could have it vaginally because I couldn't afford a C-section. So the episiotomy was really, really bad because he had to cut so much to get him out. It was worse than a C-section—I had to be on pain pills, do sitz baths [sitting in water with oils or something else soothing] … it was a rough recovery.

The lack of insurance has historically been and continues to be an obstacle to medical care for many people. Throughout the 20th century the US stood alone among advanced Western nations in its insistence on having a medical system governed by a market ideology. After the Second World War health insurance became a fringe benefit of employment, and between 1946 and 1957 the number of workers with health insurance that had been collectively bargained for by unions went from 1 million to 12 million, with more than 20 million dependents being covered (Quadagno, 2009). This left most women precariously insured, as they were not in the labor market and held insurance only as a dependent on their husband's insurance. Employer-based insurance plans also tended to omit African Americans, because most of them were employed in the more marginal sectors of the economy, such as agriculture and domestic work, where employers offered no insurance. Such insurance also excluded the elderly since, once they retired, most were unable to purchase insurance on the open market. In the early 1960s, fewer than 15 percent of people over the age of 65 had health insurance, despite being at the stage of life they were more likely to need it.

Since the passage of Medicaid and Medicare in the mid-1960s, state-sponsored insurance has been extended to the elderly and the poor, and their rates of health care utilization have grown. By 1970 a shift in the utilization of health care had occurred: people with low incomes visited doctors more often than those with high incomes, a pattern that still exists today (Cockerham, 2016). This increase in the use of health care by low-income people, however, does not mean that financial barriers to health care have been eliminated, or that the poor are receiving medical care proportionate to their needs. But it did lead to a major expansion in health care costs in the US. Medicaid and Medicare were enacted despite opposition from the AMA, but with the agreement that doctors could still charge their "usual and customary" fees. This made the government the single largest payer of medical care services as it gave doctors access to thousands of previously uninsured patients. Medical treatment for the poor and the elderly escalated, along with the rate of medical abuse and fraud among doctors, as the programs lacked price controls and proper oversight. Federal spending on health care was about $4 billion prior to Medicaid, but by 1980 it was $65.7 billion (Smedley and Stith, 2003).

Some restraints on medical reimbursements were finally put in place, resulting in a reduction in the number of doctors willing to accept Medicaid patients. The reluctance to accept Medicaid may also be related to the fact that low-income people tend to seek medical care late in the course of illness and have multiple interrelated health problems, which heightens the risk of ineffective medical treatment and possibly even being sued for malpractice if things go wrong. But some physicians do not want to deal with the administrative costs of processing their medical claims and delays in reimbursement. Treating Medicare patients—elderly patients—can also be complex, as doctors have to coordinate care with multiple other providers. One study found that primary care doctors serving Medicare patients on average have to coordinate care with 229 other doctors in 117 practices (Mechanic and McAlpine, 2010). The result is that only 42 percent of primary care doctors were found to be accepting new Medicaid patients, compared to 61 percent for Medicare and 84 percent for privately insured patients (Atherly and Mortensen, 2014).

Public funding for health care, especially for the poor, has always been a contentious issue, even more so because most of the recipients are single women and their children, and African Americans are overrepresented among them. America is a reluctant welfare state, much of it rooted in the racial heterogeneity of the population and the widespread belief that African Americans in particular are exploiting public assistance programs or are drains on the system. Political and popular fervor over the size of the welfare state escalated in the 1970s and 1980s, leading to welfare reform policies that severed the link between eligibility for public assistance and Medicaid. Welfare reform has been widely viewed as a success because millions of people left the program, but many ended up in low-paying jobs that neither lifted them out of poverty nor provided health insurance.

In 2010 more than 50 million Americans lacked health insurance, primarily those working in low-paying jobs that did not provide it as an employee benefit (Starr, 2011). My interviews with mothers revealed that many were uninsured, although their children had insurance through Medicaid eligibility. Teresa Major is a 29-year-old mother of three children and is separated from her husband. She values fitness training and health and works as a bartender and waitress, a job that pays meagerly but still disqualifies her from Medicaid:

> I am not insured; I did have Medicaid, but now my earnings keep me from it. My children are on Medicaid. I go to [a local clinic] … for the most part [the clinic] does a good job, but I cracked my top tooth and can't get an appointment. They are so booked they can't take any more appointments until after the first of the year … [but] it's not their fault they can't keep up with the patient load. Many of the doctors there do it as a service to the community.

Jackie Barnes attributes her mother's death to the lack of health insurance and the fact that her mother had a "lifelong aversion" to doctors:

> My mother was getting very small—by July we all did an intervention trying to get her to go to the doctor but she kept saying she was fine. But then she got where she couldn't go to the bathroom. She went to [the hospital], and they said she had cancer all over. She died two weeks later. She was 59 years old…. She had a lifetime aversion to doctors; I don't remember her ever going to a doctor…. Towards the end, I think it was financial and she didn't want to deal with it. I think if she had insurance she would have gone.

Another low-income mother of three, Susan Mason, is a cosmetologist who has been in her job for five years so she now has some insurance coverage, but she describes it as covering so little that it doesn't meet the requirements of the recently passed Affordable Care Act (ACA). This has meant inadequate care for her, even when she has a serious health concern:

I haven't been satisfied with the health care I've gotten. For nearly one year my whole left side was numb, I could hardly move my fingers. I continued to keep going back to the emergency room because I had met my deductible and I couldn't see a specialist. They kept trying to send me to my primary care doctor, but I don't have one. And they just told me it was stress-related, but it was—maybe not a year, but literally nine months—that my arm just tingled every day. I went to the chiropractor to pay out of pocket, which was stupid because it didn't help. At the emergency room that gave me pain pills and sent me away.

The economic recession that began in 2007 contributed immensely to the skyrocketing cost of health care provided by Medicaid, as thousands of people lost their jobs and became eligible for the programs. Medicaid enrollment grew an annual average of 6.1 percent between 2007 and 2010, with the enrollment of families a major driver in the increase (Garfield et al, 2015). Moreover, spending for acute care, which is used most often by low-income families, exceeded spending on long-term care, rising from $185.3 billion in 2007 to $284 billion in 2013 (Garfield et al, 2015). With state budgets already strained by the recession, cutting the cost of health care ranked high in the minds of policy-makers. Some research has suggested that states deliberately delay Medicaid payments to doctors, not only to keep the substantial medical funds in their accounts as long as possible, but also to curtail the use of the system (Stone, 2005).

States have also sought to reduce the cost of Medicaid by inducing more competition among health care providers. These neoliberal policies offer low-income patients the ability to choose their own provider based on quality of care and their own health needs. Consumer choice has often been a pivotal issue among those supporting privatized health care in the US, and that concept is being extended to some people who receive Medicaid. The underlying premise is that when consumers have a choice, it will spark competition among providers that lowers costs and enhances quality. But research with Medicaid beneficiaries about consumer choice revealed some interesting insights about the limitations of this market strategy for low-income African-American patients, who already have a tense relationship with their doctors (Hill et al, 2002). We found that Medicaid beneficiaries are often intimidated at the prospect of changing doctors, even when they are treated poorly. As one patient pointed out:

My blood pressure already shoots up when I go to the doctor and if I said I wanted to change doctors she [the doctor] would be insulted, and she doesn't take me seriously anyway. The last doctor before this one would get terribly mean and argumentative when I wanted to know something or had an opinion. (quoted in Hill et al, 2002: 52)

The rational choice model is essentially a middle-class concept that fails to consider how powerless and disrespected many low-income people are in dealing with medical practitioners.

Medical distrust

The poor treatment of many African Americans by medical professionals and in the medical system has generated a substantial body of literature on whether medical distrust is an obstacle to seeking medical care or accepting medical diagnoses. Trust in physicians, the belief that they will act in your best interest, has declined in general over the past 40 years with growing patient activism and consumerist attitudes. Among African Americans, however, medical mistrust may stem from a long history of racially based medical neglect, abuse, and experimentation. During the civil rights era the critique of the medical system as racist centered on widespread publicity about the use of African Americans in medical experiments. There are many instances in which the poor, institutionalized populations, and racial minorities have been used for medical experimentation, but for African Americans the Tuskegee Syphilis Study of Untreated Syphilis in the Negro Male is the best-known case. The study began in 1932 and ended in 1972, making it the longest non-therapeutic study in medical history (Freimuth et al, 2001). Publicity over the study, which received significant attention during the civil rights era, was widespread, and many people suspect that the medical system still routinely used them as guinea pigs without their knowledge (Freimuth et al, 2001).

The escalation of SCD to a major health crisis unfolded during this publicity over Tuskegee and affected the responses of some African Americans to the screening and testing for the disease. Some thought SCD was a pretext for stigmatizing and discriminating against African Americans, and others thought it was a ploy to restrict their right to have children. Explaining why she denied her daughter's sickle-cell anemia diagnosis for so long, one mother said: "The doctors were just going crazy with sickle cell. Every time a black child came in there, they would say 'sickle cell'" (quoted in Hill, 1994). Since the course of the disease is unpredictable, some mothers continued to point out that their child had none of the difficulties associated with the disease. As one mother said: "Well, nothing the doctors said was true. They said he would be sick all the time, that he would be real weak, but he's not…. Oh, and they said he was going to lose his spleen, but he hasn't lost it … so there ain't nothing wrong with him" (quoted in Hill, 1994: 165). Many mothers continued to be skeptical of the diagnosis, at least until their child's persistent sicknesses led them to accept it.

The discovery of AIDS, and especially its prevalence among African Americans and the fact that it originated in Africa, has led many black people, but especially those who are less educated and low-income, to fear that the disease is an attempt at black genocide. Although black people are significantly overrepresented among those who have and are dying from AIDS, scholars have noted that fear and medical mistrust make it difficult to recruit black people for medical trials, despite the value of understanding racial differences in drug effectiveness (Gwadz et al, 2011). Other factors also lessen the likelihood of Blacks participating in clinical trials, such as transportation and time.

In her ethnographic study of health care in a predominantly black urban community, Laurie Abraham found that many African Americans feared they were being used to test drugs or medical procedures, which made them less trustful of doctors and medical trials. For some, their fears were based on direct experience: one respondent had been incarcerated during an era when prisoners were infected with malaria in order to test new drugs. That study, conducted between 1945 and the mid-1970s, led to numerous medical reports of the impact of being infected with the bacteria, including severe abdominal pain, nausea, skin lesions, loss of appetite, and dramatic drops in blood pressure (Abraham, 1993). Prisoners nationwide have been used for all kinds of research, according to Rebecca Skloot, including testing chemical agents of warfare and X-raying testicles to see if doing so reduced sperm count. In some cases, inmates agreed to the experiments as a way of repaying for the crimes they had committed (Skloot, 2010).

Research in general reveals that many African Americans are more distrustful of medical care than Whites, although this is more the case for those who are low-income and male (Armstrong et al, 2007). Health care racism also seems to deter the utilization of preventive medical care, such as early screening for prostate cancer (Hammond et al, 2010; Shariff-Marco et al, 2010). This may make African Americans less likely to participate in medical trials or to follow physicians' recommendations; however, there is little evidence that it keeps them from seeking medical care when they are sick.

Provider–patient interactions

The effectiveness of medical care depends largely on the quality of the medical encounter and, more specifically, the provider–patient relationship. Early sociological research on the topic focused on the authority and power of doctors—based on their extensive medical training—and assumed or even prescribed deference and passivity on the part of patients. Thus, a good medical encounter consisted of an authoritative doctor and a patient who willingly obeyed the doctor's orders. Today, a model of mutual cooperation and joint participation in decision-making between doctors and patients has become the expectation, but doctors are more tolerant of this when their patients are middle-class Whites. Doctors exercise considerable discretion in how they interact and communicate with patients, and this varies based on the race and social class of the patient. Gender also matters: in the past, male physicians often treated their female patients in a patronizing and demeaning manner, and even embraced gendered medical theories that were harmful to women's health (Ehrenreich and English, 1978). Some research shows that men are more likely than women to receive advanced technological treatments such as organ transplants and coronary bypasses (Weitz, 2013). There is also evidence that white male physicians are more likely to discuss health prevention with male patients than minority or female patients (DiMatteo et al, 2009).

Race further complicates the tension between doctors and patients, especially since doctors often stereotype African-American patients as being less educated and in the lower classes. Physicians experience more social distance from black patients and describe them as being less rational, less intelligent, and less educated, regardless of their social class position (van Ryan and Burke, 2000). Regardless of payment mechanism, African Americans are less likely than Whites to receive kidney transplants or to be offered other life-preserving treatments (Xanthos et al, 2012; Weitz, 2013). Black patients with white doctors report having less opportunity for involvement in medical decision-making and report lower levels of trust and satisfaction than those with African-American doctors (DiMatteo et al, 2009). One African-American mother, for example, said:

> The doctor's major problem is that she will not wait for me to finish or listen to my explanations before rattling off judgement, eg 'you don't know anything' or 'you don't trust me, so I can't be your child's doctor.' (quoted in Hill et al, 2002: 52)

Other health care providers may have similar attitudes towards black patients. Peek and her colleagues found that fear and fatalism lowered mammogram utilization among low-income black women, but so did negative interactions with health care providers (Peek et al, 2008). The women she interviewed spoke of being treated callously by clinicians while undergoing what was already a painful screening. As one woman explained, "I'm a human being; I'm not a dog. Even dogs get treated better than us..." (Peek et al, 2008: 1849).

Most studies show that, compared to white patients, racial minority patients communicate less effectively with health care providers and receive poorer quality of health care, even when social class, health status, and insurance coverage are accounted for (Stepanikova et al, 2006). One study presented physicians with vignettes of patients who had medically ambiguous symptoms, and subliminally primed the physicians with race-ethnic data about patients. The findings revealed that physicians pursued diagnoses more aggressively for white than for black patients and were almost twice as likely to refer white patients to specialists. Some studies show that racial concordance between doctors and patients is associated with higher levels of patient satisfaction, trust, and participation in medical decision-making. But only about 22 percent of African-American patients have black physicians (Stepanikova et al, 2006).

Doctors make assumptions about their patients based on skin color, but what underlies those assumptions may be their perceptions of what Shim has called the cultural health capital of patients. She defined this as "the repertoire of cultural skills, verbal and nonverbal competencies, attitudes, and behaviors, and interactional styles, cultivated by patients and clinicians alike, that, when deployed, may result in more optimal health care relationships" (Shim, 2010: 1). Characteristics that may reflect cultural health capital include things such as health literacy, proactive attitudes, self-efficacy and mastery, and the ability to understand biomedical information. Health care providers interact differently with patients they perceive as having cultural health capital, even when that capital is embodied in their habitus rather than actually deployed. The poor, immigrants, and racial minorities are less likely than others to be perceived as having cultural health capital and, even when they do, they may have to take action to have it recognized by health care professionals.

One of my interviewees, Camille Sterner, told of her son receiving some medical treatment during a hospitalization that she was not informed about in advance. Camille, who has a doctorate in education and works as a human resources manager, was able to assert her cultural health capital only after speaking up in protest:

> Our son has a seizure disorder, a cleft cyst in his chest. And they did a few things without asking permission or consent, so I wrote a letter saying you cannot treat patients and parents this way. They sent the patient advocate, trying to clear it up. But people don't know their rights; they don't know what it is to be treated well by the health care system.

Amanda M. Gengler used the concept of cultural health capital to explore interactions between doctors and a racially diverse group of parents of children who were receiving hospital care for life-threatening illnesses. Physicians and other health care providers did not behave in an openly rude or racist way to any of their patients, but their assessment of the parents' cultural health capital shaped the ability of parents to be heard and active in decisions about medical care (Gengler, 2014). The children whose parents had high cultural health capital were often able to be "care captains" in pursuing the best treatment for their children. They mined social networks for referrals, steered the treatment, collaborated with doctors, and negotiated with insurance carriers, reaping for themselves and their children many advantages. Parents with low cultural health capital were described as "care entrusting." Physicians expected these parents to stay on the medical sidelines, to defer to medical authority, and to be passive recipients of care. Gengler argued that these micro-level doctor–patient interactions reinforce broader social inequalities and hierarchies that compromise the health care of marginalized groups.

Delores Jones, a now-widowed mother of three children, was devastated when her ten-year-old son was diagnosed with leukemia. To make matters worse, the doctors recommended that he be given chemotherapy, but also informed her and her husband that the treatment did not usually work well for African-American boys, as it tended to lead to secondary leukemia. Delores' son, in fact, had a history of responding poorly to medical interventions; for example, he experienced seizures after getting required immunization shots. She and her husband had become increasingly interested in African-based therapies and were skeptical over whether medical interventions tested on and used for white people were appropriate for African Americans. Their doubts were strengthened when the doctor warned them that chemotherapy did not work well for black boys, and they had one question for the doctor: "What do we have to do to get him out of here?" They checked their son out against medical advice but, as Delores explained:

> They [the doctors] got right with the authorities; the sheriff was at our door, threatening to remove him from our home. [My husband] had friends, he got a medical doctor to testify for us ... arguing with him the fact that the usual treatment often doesn't work for us ... we were genetically different in so many ways.... We went to court and I guess you could say we lost....

Delores is convinced that the alternative therapy they were using was working, but they were forced under threat of having her son removed from the home to take him for chemotherapy. After two years of treatment, her son developed secondary leukemia and died—an outcome doctors had told them was likely. Leukemia is a serious disease and the medical system is correct in intervening to ensure children get the best treatment possible. Still, Delores was devastated by not being able to even discuss the possibility of alternative treatment with her physician, especially given their own admission that chemotherapy was not very effective in treating black boys.

Organization of medicine

Dutton argued that the strongest factor affecting the low utilization of medical care among the poor was the organization of medicine, such as the lack of adequate health care facilities in poor neighborhoods, long waits for medical care, the lack of continuity of care, and often inappropriate and impersonal care. The quality of care factors are largely influenced by whether a person has private, public, or no health insurance, and whether they are accessing care in the public or private sector of the health care system. African Americans and Whites are almost equally like to have health insurance; however, 65 percent of Whites have private insurance, compared to 45 percent of Blacks (Cockerham, 2016). African Americans are only slightly more likely than Whites to have no health insurance at all, but are two times more likely to rely on public health insurance (Medicaid) than Whites. Thus, they are likely to receive medical care that differs greatly in availability and quality.

These dramatic differences in medical care were illustrated in a study by Lutfey and Freese, who compared treatment of diabetes patients in two different medical settings. They found significant differences between the organization of health services and the quality of care one received in the private versus the public sector of the health care system. The predominantly white patients at Park Clinic were affluent and well insured, and those as County Clinic were mostly lower- and working-class and racial minority; more than 40 percent were uninsured. Park Clinic patients received treatment in the private sector of the health care system, where they had shorter waits for their appointments, consulted with doctors rather than medical interns and students, received superior educational resources for managing their diabetes, and experienced greater continuity of care. Since they were able to see the same doctor with each visit, an important element of medical care, Park Clinic patients built strong relationships and rapport with their doctors; the doctors often knew quite a bit about their patients' work and family lives (Lutfey and Freese, 2005). Patients receiving care at County Clinic had exactly the opposite experience, exemplifying what Dutton called system barriers to care.

The emergency room care dilemma

The overuse of emergency room care has been a perpetual issue in the US, as it is one of the most expensive forms of medical care. Emergency room care exemplifies one of the structural barriers to care discussed by Dutton. People often seek emergency room care because of an acute condition and lack of alternative sources of medical care. The Emergency Medical Treatment and Labor Act of 1986 prohibited turning people away from emergency rooms without a medical screening exam, even if such exams lead to hospitalization (Fontenot, 2014). As Mark Downs, a 60-year-old married man, who has held a series of jobs that pay just above the poverty level, said:

> I don't have a permanent care doctor, so I have to go to the
> hospital emergency room, and take whatever care I can get.
> I have to go there—but not just for a cold or something.
> But any major problem, I go through the emergency room.

I've had a couple of bad experiences with doctors there ...
they won't listen to you.

In other cases, physicians may send their patients to emergency rooms
simply because they are unavailable to provide care on the weekends
or in the evenings. One mother with a chronically ill daughter noted
her frustration with this care:

> When I have a medical emergency, he [the doctor] sends
> me straight to the hospital, which really upsets me because
> the emergency room doctors don't have a case file on her.
> Not to mention I have to get a referral every time I go to
> the ER which, by the way, the doctor occasionally tends to
> forget to call the hospital. (quoted in Hill et al, 2002: 51)

Many people who arrive in emergency rooms, even those with
severe injuries, face overcrowding, long waits, a lack of privacy, and
questionable care. One sickle-cell anemia patient described having to
wait several hours to be treated during a severe pain crisis:

> I was screaming, I was hurting, and I said 'Somebody needs
> to do something,' because I was throwing up. I was having
> a fever. I felt like I was going to faint and they were like
> 'Just give us two more hours'....

Such experiences were common among other adults in this sickle-cell
anemia focus group (Ciribassi and Patil, 2016). In fact, these authors
cited research showing that sickle-cell patients who are in severe pain
waited longer in emergency rooms to get pain medication than white
patients with a similar painful disease (for example, renal colic).

Emergency rooms in large urban areas are often filled with people
needing care for maladies ranging from elevated fevers to gunshot
wounds, often exacerbated by the AIDS crises, drug-related crimes,
homelessness, and mental illness (Abraham, 1993). Many emergency
rooms are poorly staffed and lack adequate medical equipment; foreign
medical school graduates who are less likely to be board-certified and
are less knowledgeable about the complexities of the US health care
system or the cultural diversity of the population comprise a significant
number of the doctors (Smedley and Stith, 2003). One young black
man, explaining why he tried to avoid getting medical care, said:
"Every time I go to the hospital.... I'm getting a foreign doctor who
barely speaks English and they treat me like a young black hoodlum

so ... why even go?" (quoted in Ravenell et al, 2008). Still, for some patients, the emergency room means getting treatment in hours instead of waiting weeks for a doctor's appointment and not being asked for a co-payment or being turned away due to lack of insurance.

Conclusion

Deborah Stone has argued that the market ideology is the major obstacle to equity in the US health care system, and has fueled racial fears that reduce the likelihood that disadvantaged people across racial lines can mobilize for change. Dominant discourses on consumer choice and states' rights often mask and perpetuate racial tensions and health disparities. As Stone has written:

> Market principles create, perpetuate, and intensify racial and ethnic disparities. Market ideology not only justifies racial and ethnic disparities in health care, it allows racism to continue under the cover of economic justifications. (Stone, 2005: 66)

Access to medical care will likely expand as the provisions of the ACA are enacted. The political furor over the Act has bought to the fore racially divisive politics and also highlighted the power of market ideologies and notions of consumer choice. Many Americans believe that the US has the best health care system in the world, have little knowledge of significant inequities in care, and believe that those without health insurance should simply purchase it in the open market. But employment-based insurance, which once hid the real cost of medical care from consumers, has now become much less available. Today, slightly more than half of all employers offer health insurance, and many of those policies are shifting more of the costs to consumers (Fontenot, 2014). Although it is unlikely to happen in the near future, the ACA requirement for reform in the health insurance industry has the potential of eliminating many inequities in access to medical care.

Part Three
Health and families

Families are important entities in shaping the health of their members. Historically, families were the major source of medical care (see Chapter Two) and, with the increase in chronic illnesses, much medical caregiving has been transferred back to families. But the impact of families on health extends far beyond caring for the sick: the family is the oldest social institution in existence and evolved to enhance the survival of its members, usually by organizing work, reproduction, and sexuality. Modern families have lost many of their traditional functions, but still have the important role of socializing children. Moreover, they are the locus of our most formative and intimate social relationships. In that sense, families influence our health more profoundly than medical care, and their influence is mediated by structural inequalities. This part of the book looks at African-American health in family context.

Although black families are diverse in social class and family structure—and always have been—they share a legacy of racial and economic oppression that continues to undermine intimate and marital relationships, family stability, and the ability to successfully socialize children. For centuries African Americans were not only forced to prioritize work over family, but to endure the violation of practically every religious and moral principle pertaining to family life. After slavery ended, black families continued to be stigmatized for failing to conform to dominant family norms but were also penalized for trying to do so, especially when their efforts compromised white control of their labor (Jones, 1985; Dill, 1988).

The final three chapters of the book examine African-American families within the context of the post-industrial economy that began to emerge in the 1970s—less than a decade after the gains of the civil rights era. This economic decline has had an adverse effect on families of all races; many have experienced job loss, declining and stagnant wages, less social mobility, and the loss of worker benefits such as health insurance and pensions. As with most transitions, however, the new economy has disproportionately affected those who were already on the margins, those who lacked the resources and skills to reposition themselves in the new economy. African Americans were overrepresented among those on the economic margins; thus, the evolution of the post-industrial economy had a profound impact on their families and communities, especially in terms of nonmarriage, non-marital childbirth, violence, and the use of illicit drugs. The policy response to the crisis has been the implementation of punitive welfare and drug policies, the latter of which have led to mass incarceration and a resurgence of overt expressions of racism. This has affected African Americans across social class boundaries, as they cope with low rates of marriage, fractured families, and the imprisonment of family members.

The negative health consequences of illicit drug use and mass incarceration are multiplied by the post-industrial economy's corrosive impact on intimate relationships and marriage. Scholars have described a "love and trouble" tradition between black men and women sparked by their inability to conform to conventional gender ideologies, resulting in inequalities in access to love and intimacy. Yet loving relationships are known to enhance health, while transient, exploitative, and conflictual relationships diminish it. They also make it difficult to form the kinds of families in which children can thrive and achieve. Children are adversely affected by family instability and transitions, the loss of parents through separation and divorce, poverty, and the broader social context in which they live. These topics are the focus of this part of the book, and this introduction provides a broader theoretical and historical context for understanding the connection between families, the economy, and health.

Historical context of families in transition

One of the earliest observations of sociologists was that massive social changes disrupted social institutions, altered human behaviors, and redefined cultural values. Theorizing the impact of the rise of the industrial economy in the 1800s, Émile Durkheim, one of the founders of sociology, pointed out that such change diminished social integration and cohesion among people. This often resulted in a sense of normlessness, or anomie, in which people no longer felt bound to social rules and were more likely to engage in deviant behaviors, or even suicide. Major changes in the economy can also adversely affect health. The evolution of 19th-century industrial capitalism sparked a crisis of sickness and death, especially among those in the working class.

The more recent transition to a post-industrial society has resulted in significant job loss, stagnant wages, and declining mobility and, during the 1970s and 1980s, elevated rates of serious chronic illness—both mental and physical—across Western societies (Brenner, 1987).

Economic transitions have a major impact on families, as their resiliency and ability to meet the needs of their members depends largely on the nature of dominant economy. In the agricultural economy of colonial America, survival often meant living in multigenerational households, the joint participation of men and women in productive labor, high rates of fertility, and the transfer of property and work skills from parents to children. The transition to an industrial economy challenged this family model and caused so much disruption that many surmised the family was becoming extinct (Cherlin, 2013). After some decades, the industrial economy stabilized, workers gained better pay, and new family and gender ideologies emerged. The breadwinner-homemaker family became the dominant cultural ideal, although it did not become the most common family structure until the 1940s and 1950s, an era often referred to as the "golden age of the family."

The post-war affluence and extensive government investments in housing, education, and other infrastructural improvements greatly aided in supporting the male wage-earner family and making the US a middle-class society (Coontz, 2005). African-American families experienced some of the benefits of the new economic affluence, but the legacy of slavery and continuing racial segregation made it impossible for many to conform to the male wage-earner family model. Slavery influenced the development of black families by forbidding legal marriages, separating and selling husbands, wives, and children, negating the parental rights of enslaved parents, and encouraging and forcing casual and often nonconsensual sexual relationships. In addition to fostering sickness and death, slavery brutalized black bodies and minds, and the sharecropping system that replaced it provided little opportunity for a better life. Racial hostility and efforts to control the sexuality and labor of African Americans resulted in enduring racial stereotypes that affect popular perceptions of black people, as well as their own identities and behaviors. These racial stereotypes cast black men and women as sexual and moral menaces to society—women as sexually irresponsible single mothers who emasculate men and rely on the state for economic support, and men as criminally inclined sexual predators who are prone to evading the responsibilities of work and family life.

These racialized gender stereotypes have had an immense impact on African Americans as they struggled to achieve stable marriages and families. Moreover, they re-emerge with a vengeance when black people are seen as threatening the welfare of racially dominant groups—and this intensifies racial discrimination and hostility and leads to other adverse consequences. The massive migration of black people from the South to the North during the early decades of the 20th century offers one example. Between 1870 and 1950, 3.2 million non-white people—mostly African Americans—migrated northward in search of better job opportunities. The early black migrants often had intact families and more education than those who came later, but they still faced significant racial barriers to finding employment—men more than women, as the latter typically accepted domestic work. Still, black migration created a panic, especially among white ethnic groups who felt their economic and social status was being jeopardized by the arrival of thousands of new people. One result was the "whitening" of European minority ethnic groups, as they coalesced to distance themselves from Blacks (Muller, 2012). Another was a renewed effort to criminalize black men. Focusing on the intense policing and arrest of black men in Chicago, one of the major destinations of black migrants, Muller found that the rate of nonwhite incarceration nearly tripled between 1880 and 1950, even as the incarceration of white men fell. By 1922, the city's Commission on Race Relations concluded:

> The testimony is practically unanimous that Negros are much more liable to arrest than whites, since police officers share in the general public opinion that Negroes "are more criminal than whites," and also feel that there is little risk of trouble in arresting Negroes, while greater care must be exercised in arresting whites. (quoted in Muller, 2012)

This criminalization followed a pattern found in southern states where, after the abolition of slavery, black men were often imprisoned for minor offenses, either to secure their labor in work camps (Britton, 2011) or to disenfranchise them from voting (Holloway, 2014). Incarceration removed black men from families and the paid labor force, while also compromising their citizenship rights.

In addition to the adverse consequences of slavery, northward migration had a destabilizing effect on African-American families, according to E. Franklin Frazier, a notable black sociologist who was among a handful studying black families in the early decades of the 20th century. Many black migrants obtained gainful employment, many did not, and rates of marital failure, nonmarital childbearing, and welfare dependence soared. Most scholars focused on black families who failed to conform to the married-couple, male wage-earner family model, concluding that black families were dysfunctional (Frazier, 1948, 1957 [1939]). In fact, the dominant theory was that the legacy of slavery had practically destroyed black families—a theory that sparked decades of heated debates when reiterated in the infamous Moynihan Report of the 1960s (Moynihan, 1965). Moynihan argued that slavery in the US had been "indescribably worse than, any recorded servitude, ancient or modern," (1965: 15) and was responsible for the major problem facing African Americans: single-mother and father-absent families. Issued amid the civil rights movement and the revival of cultural studies, the Moynihan Report was refuted by revisionist research on black families that emphasized their historic stability and cultural strengths (Gutman, 1976).

Within a decade, however, this new cultural perspective was beginning to ring hollow: while many African-American families had experienced significant economic mobility and were thriving, the post-industrial economy was taking a toll on thousands of other black families. This pattern of social class polarization mirrored that found in the dominant society, where the new post-industrial economy was challenging the ideology of the male wage-earner family. The percentage of the economy based on manufacturing fell from 40 percent during the post-Second World War era to 8.1 percent by 2010, with more than 8 million manufacturing jobs lost between 1979 and 2012 (Wysong et al, 2014).

The post-industrial economy continues to transform conventional families. The dual-income family has become the norm, and women are demanding more equity in the domestic area and equal pay in the labor market. Men are more likely than in the past to attitudinally—if not behaviorally—support gender equality in the home. The rise of jobs paying meager wages and joblessness has challenged traditional notions of masculinity, as men struggle to redefine their place in the family. Marriage rates have declined and gender tensions have escalated, especially among those in the working and lower classes. The decline in job opportunities for men has coincided with a historic rise in the rate of male incarceration. In 2008, the Pew Institute reported that 1 in every 100 adults in the US was behind bars—by far the highest rate of incarceration of any Western nation

This economic downturn has especially affected African-American families, many of which were already struggling to survive. Blacks have experienced the sharpest decline in employment and marriage, and the highest rates of incarceration, with serious health consequences for families, communities, and children.

FIVE

Economic decline and incarceration

Mary Nash grew up in a stable, two-parent, working-class family, married at an early age, and had two sons. She divorced and remarried her husband, only to divorce him again, so for the most part she raised her sons as a single mother. Mary still managed to attend college and earn a bachelor's degree, thus achieving some socioeconomic mobility, but that did not protect her or her sons against the homicide and drug epidemic that spiked during the 1980s. One of her sons was murdered and the other one is in jail, awaiting trial on a drugs offense. Speaking of this experience, Mary said:

> My son was murdered due to street crime. He wasn't hanging out on the street—he had his own place and was working [on a job]. They [the police] found him shot—they found his body at the back of [a park]. They didn't do anything, because it was homicide. At least they never got back with me. Well, they did want to interview me, my son, and my ex-when it first happened, but I don't want to know what happened to him. His brother took it pretty hard and he uses that to explain whatever goes wrong in his life.

The stresses of life have taken a toll on Mary's health. She is dealing with fibroid tumors and is being treated for osteoporosis and hepatitis C. She has no idea how she got the latter and fought the diagnosis for a while, but finally accepted treatment when her physician offered to put her in clinical trials, meaning she would not have to pay for it. Mary is also stressed over dealing with her remaining son, a 32-year-man who has never been able find a stable life for himself:

> Dealing with my son is stressful. He stays in trouble. He is locked up now in jail and is supposed to be sentenced this month for drugs. Our system doesn't do a good job of finding out what really happened. They just want to put our men away.

After 30 years of escalating rates of incarceration, the tendency of society to "put our men away" has finally emerged as a major social and political issue. In her important book, the *New Jim Crow: Mass incarceration in the age of colorblindness*, Michelle Alexander details the policing practices and policies that have landed thousands of African Americans, especially men, in prison, often for minor drugs offenses (Alexander, 2010). Skyrocketing rates of incarceration unfolded in the context of the economic decline that began in the 1970s and resulted in high rates of unemployment, nonmarriage, drug trafficking, crime, and homicide in black neighborhoods. Although some African-American families were affected by the transition more than others, the consequences of it have cut across social class and generational boundaries. Racism and segregation have challenged the viability of black families for centuries, but their decline in the post-civil rights era—an era that promised new opportunities and greater support for racial equality—was especially disheartening. It challenged revisionist scholarship and the cultural perspective on African-American families, both of which emphasized their strengths and ability to survive. Theories of black family pathology were reignited, as were racial stereotypes that described African Americans as inherently immoral, criminally inclined, and more prone to welfare than work.

Chaos, violence, and drug trafficking seemed to reign in many black neighborhoods, capturing extensive media attention and alarm over the growing "black underclass." Marriage rates plummeted, nonmarital childbirth became the statistical norm, and black children landed in foster care in unprecedented numbers. Sociologist William J. Wilson advanced the thesis that the post-industrial economy, which had caused massive job loss among young African-American men, was the major factor in the problems facing inner-city communities. By the mid-1970s, low-income and working-class black men were much more likely to be unemployed than they were in the 1950s. Policy-makers, however, often blamed the problem on the bad behavior of African Americans, arguing that they simply refused to abide by mainstream cultural norms. For many, the solution was to discipline black people through punitive welfare and penal policies.

The impact of the economic decline of the 1970s has had far-reaching consequences for many African Americans. It bears pointing out that this economic decline has affected people of all races, especially those in the working- and lower-classes, making it more difficult for them to marry or earn wages sufficient to support their families and resulting in higher rates of incarceration. African Americans have simply been affected more broadly because of their historic economic marginality and the backlash of racial hostilities sparked by the declining status of white working-class families. The popular stereotype of African-American single mothers as "welfare queens" was the major impetus for welfare reform, and African-American men have been disproportionately affected by drug laws enacted in the 1980s, with many imprisoned for nonviolent or drugs-related offenses. While the overall rate of incarceration was 1 per 100 for American adults, the rate for white men was 1 for every 106, compared to 1 for every 15 black men and 1 in 9 for those between the ages of 20 and 34. Drugs-related incarceration has affected thousands of black families and has significantly impacted their health.

The "crack epidemic"

Robert Merton applied the concept of anomie (or "normlessness") to crime, explaining that crime arises when people share the societal goals, but lack the means to achieve those goals. This offers a framework for explaining how diminished job prospects among young African Americans coincided with escalating rates of the use and sale of illicit drugs, especially crack cocaine. Cocaine trafficking expanded in the US during the late 1970s, but for political reasons was not initially seen as a social problem (Logan, 1999). Crack cocaine, which first appeared in 1981, was the result of an effort to increase profits from the drug by making cocaine "rocks" that could be sold on the streets. Crack cocaine was easily accessible, highly addictive, and could be sold in affordable quantities; thus, it quickly became a way for low-income and poor men to earn money and, to some extent, status. The crack epidemic led to high rates of drug dependence, violence, sickness, and early death among African Americans in general, and brought to the fore longstanding racialized gender stereotypes.

For African-American men it reinforced stereotypes of their innate criminality and resulted in high rates of violence, homicide, and incarceration. Drug trafficking has often been thought of as an economically lucrative alternative for young men, especially more appealing than joblessness and menial low-wage work. But only a handful of those peddling drugs actually earned wages sufficient to support themselves; most peddlers earned little, and ran a high risk of violence and early death in return for their efforts. The high rate of homicide among young African-American men led some to refer to them as a "vanishing species," a term that quickly became controversial. Nevertheless, the death rate among young black men spiraled—as did their seeming lack of concern over dying young. Black men have the lowest life expectancy of any racial group, much of it related to homicide: the current homicide rate for black males between the ages of 15 to 29 is 75 for every 100,000, compared to 4 for every 100,000 white males (Martin et al, 2015).

Drug trafficking did, however, offer some young men an avenue to masculinity they could not attain through more traditional means, such as power or career success. When I interviewed Ronnie, he was 40 years old and had long since grown tired of life on the street and of selling drugs. But he said that doing so had made him feel important and respected. Practically everyone in his part of town knew him as "the man" who could "hook you up," and he enjoyed the "cat and mouse" aspect of dodging the police. In addition to gaining status, the epidemic of drugs occurred in the context of a distinct shift in black cultural norms aimed at asserting patriarchal power and refuting notions that black men had been emasculated by strong, independent black women. Many young black men acquiesced to norms of displaying masculinity through displays of violence or "cool pose"—a tough image that masks emotions and projects a willingness to fight or die over even minor conflicts (Majors and Billson, 1992). Misogynistic rap music proliferated, containing invectives against black women and urging their subordination, even through violence. Intimate partner violence was not invented during the economic crisis of the 1970s and 1980s, but it certainly became more prevalent and visible.

When I interviewed Mildred Harris, she was 46 years old and, after many attempts, had finally successfully completed a drug rehabilitation program. Mildred had been in a relationship for more than 20 years with "the man of her dreams,"—a smart, handsome man who was well-known in the neighborhood and always had money. Mildred said she did not initially relate this to being involved with drugs, but over the course of the relationship she not only became addicted to crack, but also the victim of multiple serious beatings from a man who often explained he was trying to teach her how to be the "right kind" of woman. In some cases, they were both "high" when the conflict ensued, and it often involved being threatened with a gun. In one of those instances, Mildred said:

> I tried to push the gun out of his hand and we really fought over that gun. And I got really beat up, just because he wanted to teach me that I was a woman, and I should learn to never fight a man ... for any reason. So I got beat up for stepping out of a 'woman's place,' whatever that is.

Mildred said that trips to the emergency room became so common that the doctors knew her by name, and often asked when she was going to get out of this relationship. She continued to suffer serious physical abuse—in one episode of violence losing most of her teeth—but for years told herself that she was a "strong enough woman" to make the relationship work. Although she has been out of the relationship for years now (her partner was sent to prison), she still suffers myriad health challenges related to the years of drug abuse and intimate partner violence.

"Crack babies:" the new narrative on deficient black mothers

The extent to which African-American women were involved in the sale of drugs remains to be fully explored, but by most counts their participation was mostly as accessories to the activities of the men they were involved with. There is much evidence, however, that they were victims of the crack epidemic. By the early 1990s, black women were more likely than women of other racial groups to have used crack cocaine, and they accounted for 40 percent of all drugs-related emergency room visits and 30 percent of all drugs-related deaths (Collins, 1996).

Low-income single mothers were especially likely to fall prey to the drug epidemic, and were being blamed for the escalating number of health impairments, cognitive defects, and behavioral problems among black children. At least 30 states passed laws calling for the arrest and incarceration of pregnant women whose prenatal tests revealed they were smoking crack cocaine or new mothers with babies who were diagnosed as drug-addicted (Roberts, 1997). By 1989, 82 percent of Americans agreed that a pregnant woman who used crack cocaine and addicted her unborn child to the drug should go to jail for child abuse. This added to the growing number of incarcerated women, which grew fivefold between 1980 and 2000. By 1980, African-American women—who comprised only 12 percent of the female population—made up 46 percent of female inmates in state prisons and 39 percent of female inmates in federal prison (Solinger, 2005). Researchers found that black women were more likely than white women to be prosecuted and to receive a long prison sentence, although there was little evidence that their drug use was significantly higher (Bush-Baskette, 1998).

In 1989 a low-income African-American woman named Jennifer Johnson became the first person to be convicted of giving birth to an infant who had been prenatally exposed to drugs. She was found guilty of having delivered a controlled substance to a minor, and received a 15-year sentence—1 year to be spent in prison and 14 on probation. Johnson's probation included drug treatment, random drug-testing, and vocational training, and required her to inform her probation officer if she ever intended to become pregnant again (Logan, 1999).

For two decades medical professionals, political leaders, and the popular media focused on the "crack cocaine epidemic" that was seen as devastating low-income, urban neighborhoods. Health care workers were quick to claim that newborn infants who had any medical issue were victims of drug abuse. For example, a nurse in the neonatal intensive care unit of an Oakland, California hospital located in a low-income black area claimed that at least 20 percent of all babies were being born addicted to drugs and described them this way:

> They can't be cuddled like normal babies. Often their arm and legs, even their necks, are rigid. They don't fall into normal sleep patterns.... They cry incessantly. Their stomach cramps make them want to eat but their digestive systems cannot handle food. What we watch to prevent is a seizure. We hope to minimize brain damage. (quoted in *The Economist*, 1989: 28)

The narrative surrounding crack babies was highly racialized, with significant implications for the reproductive rights of African-American mothers. Crack babies were always assumed to be black babies borne by irresponsible black mothers, who not only neglected their children but would even sell them into prostitution for drug money (Glenn, 2014). In a critical summary of evidence from numerous studies, Logan catalogued the litany of health problems these infants were presumed to suffer as a result of their mother's irresponsible behavior, including premature birth, low birth weight, neonatal strokes, growth retardation, cerebral hemorrhaging, cardiac abnormalities, unpredictable mood swings and "high-pitched cat-like crying," among other things. Many claimed that these babies were unlikely to be able to learn to read or to concentrate, and would be prone to violent and destructive behaviors. Crack babies were seen as polluted and impure and as a liability to society and to taxpayers.

By 1990, however, cocaine-related admissions to hospitals were beginning to decline although, as one article pointed out, "politicians have been reluctant to accept that their pet hysteria is now passed" (*The Economist*, 1990: 28). In 2001 a meta-analysis of research called into question the whole idea of crack babies, concluding that the concept had no scientific basis (Glenn, 2014). For example, many of these studies failed to verify the type of drugs the infant had been exposed to, to explore their long-term impact, or to consider the extent to which the symptoms of the infants were related to poverty, poor maternal nutrition, stressful prenatal conditions, or the lack of prenatal care. More recently, research has found that while cocaine use among pregnant women is by no means inconsequential, the evidence that it causes long-term physical or mental problems for children is limited.

Longitudinal research has found no significant influence of prenatal exposure to cocaine on the IQ or language development of children, and argued that the issue was more of moral crisis than a health crisis (Okie, 2009). Nevertheless, the crack babies narrative helped derail revisionist scholarship on the strengths of African-American families and the ability of mothers, especially those who were unmarried, to successfully raise their children. Black women have historically been praised as "mammies" who could tend to the needs of white children and families, but vilified as the antithesis of the good mother when it came to raising their own children (Hill, 2008). The crack epidemic reinvigorated notions of deficient black mothers, with many calling for prison, the loss of maternal custody rights, and even the creation of orphanages for the children of mothers who have used crack cocaine.

The long arm of the drug epidemic

Camille Sterner is a married, 39-year-old mother of two who recently earned her doctorate degree. When I interviewed her—just a few months ago—she had recently returned from the funeral of a second aunt who had died from drug-related illnesses. Drug use permeates the community and culture of her family. She said:

I have family members who have dealt with drugs and alcohol addiction. Quite honestly, it's such that I would probably say that my family has addictive personalities—it's like once we start going in a general direction, it's hard to change from that. My mother is one of eight siblings, and two of her siblings died from drug-related issues. My two aunts who died, they were not raised in the same house with my mother ... they lived with their mother and it was the circumstances they grew up in—I'm not saying they didn't have a choice, but every single one of them has struggled with drug addiction. I just got back from my last aunt's funeral.... The circumstances and environment in the community they live in doesn't lead to any other escape except that [drug use]. My cousins who are 6 and 7 or so, it's all around them—the relatives are using it, their friends are using it. It's normal for them—they don't have any hope of coming out of this situation of addiction.... This is not deviant for them, it's normal.

The drug epidemic has resulted in the placement of many African-American children in foster care, either with relatives or non-relatives. One 73-year-old grandmother, so out of touch with her drug-addicted daughter that she did not know she had given birth to a son, recalled receiving a phone call from her daughter one day:

She said 'I got kicked out of my apartment. I don't have a job. I'm living out of my car. Family Services is about to take [my son] away from me. Would you come get him?' I said 'Absolutely.' I didn't prepare myself at all ... and once I got [my grandson] here, I knew I was in trouble. This poor little baby was sick and he cried all the time. (Letiecq et al, 2008: 1002)

The crack epidemic, high rates of crime and violence, the decline of marriage, and the rise of nonmarital childbearing and welfare dependency among black women roused political controversy but few policies targeting the issue of racial disparities in employment and opportunities. Instead, a highly racialized discourse about nonmarital pregnancy, welfare, and illicit drugs emerged. Arguing that skyrocketing out-of-wedlock births were ripping apart our nation's social fabric (McCormack, 2005), conservative politicians claimed that generous welfare policies were leading women to choose welfare over marriage and employment. Many saw curtailing the public sector of the welfare system as the answer to the problem, and efforts to do so began with widespread accusations that welfare fraud was rampant and a few federally sponsored programs designed to move mothers from welfare to work. Although the programs received considerable publicity and stirred some debate over whether mothers of young children should be required to work outside of the home, they overall fell short of providing poor mothers with the job skills, education, or resources they needed to enter the labor market (Seccombe, 2007). Nevertheless, thousands of mothers lost their eligibility for Aid to Families with Dependent Children and, during the 1980s, federal and state funding for subsidized housing, nutritional planning, food stamps, and family planning was sharply curtailed.

The 1980s also saw a revival of the "war on drugs" rhetoric, a concept that had first been articulated in the 1970s. Declaring that the crack epidemic was threatening American values and undercutting its institutions, President Reagan called for more attention from the media and medical authorities to publicize the problem, and they responded with literally hundreds of articles on the drug addicton crisis. With the passage of the Anti-Drug Abuse Act, federal spending on the nation's drug problem escalated from $200 million in 1970 to $13 billion in 1992, with most of the money spent on law enforcement (Roberts, 1997). The Act created a 100 to one disparity in the sentencing between those persons convicted of possessing or trafficking crack cocaine rather than powdered cocaine, which led to more drug convictions and longer prison sentences for African Americans. A person convicted of possessing five grams of crack cocaine—the drug most common among black people—received a minimum mandatory sentence of five years, but one had to possess 500 grams of powder cocaine for such a sentence to be imposed. Thus, as the rate of violent crime declined significantly during the 1990s, the rate of incarceration skyrocketed (Alexander, 2010; Coates, 2015).

Scholars have argued that the lower rate of unemployment in the US during the 1980s and 1990s was directly related to the expansion of the penal system, which, in essence, became a strategy for controlling a potentially restive population of unemployed men (Western and Beckett, 1999). By the early 1990s, the nation was spending $41 billion on unemployment benefits and related services, but $91 billion on the courts, police, and prisons. The prison population increased 300 percent between 1980 and 1996, with 1.63 million people in prison—disproportionately young black men. By 1995, 7 percent of black men were incarcerated and one in three of all young black men were under some kind of court-ordered supervision. In 1979, 6 percent of prison inmates had been convicted of nonviolent drug offenses, but by 1994 that figure had risen to 30 percent.

Incarceration and health

The impact of incarceration on the health of inmates and their families has been the focus of a growing amount of research. A few have suggested that those who are incarcerated—mostly the poor and racial minorities—may gain better access to health care than they previously had. Many people who enter prison come from family backgrounds with significant disadvantages, including food insecurity, childhood neglect and abuse, and homelessness. The medical exams given upon entry to prison overall reveal high rates of acute and chronic illnesses. There is also a high rate of psychiatric disorders among inmates, the origins of which often lie in childhood or adolescent trauma (Schnittker et al, 2012). Yet research finds that disease is more prevalent among inmates than among their nonincarcerated same-age peers, and that a history of incarceration strongly increases the chances of severe health limitations after release (Schnittker and John, 2007). Most research, in fact, shows that incarceration has an adverse impact on health through multiple mechanisms. For starters, state and federal budgets are too strained to provide much beyond the most basic medical care to inmates.

Incarceration and adjustment to prison life are major life transitions that produce stress and increase the likelihood of stress-related illness. Health has been shown to be related to one's ability (or perceived ability) to control one's life and participate in society, which is severely diminished by incarceration. Prisons are total institutions that control virtually every aspect of one's life, from wearing prison clothing to regulating meal and bed times. Scholars have long argued that prisoners undergo a process of prisonization, which diminishes the former identities of inmates, makes them anonymous members of a subordinate group, and requires them to develop new behaviors (Comfort, 2008).

Being in prison significantly increases one's exposure to a wide range of infectious diseases, including tuberculosis, hepatitis B, hepatitis C, HIV, AIDS, and other sexually transmitted diseases. One study found that 20 percent of people in the US who are infected with HIV pass through correctional institutions in a given year, and outbreaks of contagious diseases such as tuberculosis have been directly traced to prisons (Massoglia, 2008a, 2008b). Prisons expose inmates to a variety of living conditions and survival mechanisms that adversely affect their health. Violence is prolific in prisons and the source of much physical harm and psychological distress. Prisoners are subjected to inhumane and violent treatment at the hands of guards and other inmates, sometimes leading to death, and the possibility of such mistreatment is the source of chronic stress for the families of inmates. The abuse and/or beating to death of inmates by prison guards, as in the 2010 case of Leonard Strickland, costs the prison system millions of dollars in legal suits, and points to the need for more monitoring of the system (Deitch and Mushlin, 2016).

The number of inmates held in solitary confinement has soared in recent decades, despite significant research pointing to its severe health consequences. Prisoners are often held in solitary confinement for prolonged periods of time for minor infractions of rules, effectively deprived of sunlight, proper ventilation, decent food, and human contact (Cloud et al, 2015). Suicide rates are high in prison, but five times higher for those held in solitary confinement than for other inmates. Moreover, prisoners who are released directly from solitary confinement back to the community have much higher rates of violence and recidivism than those released from the general prison population (Cloud et al, 2015).

The health of women who are in prison deteriorates over time. Aday and Krabill (2011) examined women who were aging in prison and found they experienced high rates of mental health problems. About two-thirds of the female inmates they studied described their health as either "fair" or "poor." Many suffered from constant physical pain—often the result of drug abuse or the sexual or physical abuse they experienced before incarceration. To compound the problem many also are physically or sexually abused by correctional officers, and they receive poor gynecological and obstetrical care (Comfort, 2008).

Incarceration not only affects the health of felons but also that of their families, a fact that is often referred to as collateral damage. About half of incarcerated men describe themselves as being in committed relationships, and their partners experience heightened stress along with the mental and physical effects of their incarceration. They experience more uncertainty and social isolation, and have a higher risk of major depressive episodes and life dissatisfaction (Wildeman et al, 2012). The families of incarcerated men often have to deal with cycles of separation and reimprisonment, and visiting their incarcerated partners takes a toll on their meager resources. Families and especially intimate partners spend money on court fees, lawyers, telephone calls, visiting, and often food and clothing for their incarcerated loved one.

Almost one in every four women and two in every five black women are related to someone who is incarcerated (Diuguid, 2016).

Comfort has argued that the women who have relationships with incarcerated men become "quasi inmates" who experience secondary prisonization, as their relationships unfold under the watchful eyes of prison guards (Comfort et al, 2005; Comfort, 2008). They live with restrictive visiting guidelines, including rules about what they can wear and how much physical contact they can have with their partners. Many also endure inexplicably long waiting times for their partners to be brought in to see them. This takes a toll on their health and that of their unborn children—mothers who have incarcerated partners are much less likely to have healthy babies. Research finds a 40 percent increase in infant mortality among mothers of incarcerated partners (Wildeman et al, 2012).

Parental incarceration also adversely affects the lives of thousands of African-American children. A black child born in 1978 faced a 1:7 chance of having their father sent to prison before their 14th birthday compared to 1:50 for white children. By 2000, 1 million black children had a father in prison, half of whom were living with the child before incarceration (Coates, 2015), and about 25 percent of young African Americans will have had a father in prison at some point in their lives (Wakefield and Wildeman, 2014). For many, an imprisoned father is more than a missing caregiver or breadwinner, but someone you may have watched being handcuffed or wrestled to the ground, or had to visit by looking through prison bars or windows. Needless to say, the process of arrest and incarceration can be traumatizing and stressful for children; not surprisingly, they experience stigma and demonstrate more externalizing or problematic behaviors that require clinical intervention, such as hyperactivity, aggression, and delinquency (Wildeman et al, 2012). The odds of homelessness for children may also increase, at least in some poor urban areas, and those who end up in homeless shelters are exposed to higher rates of abuse and disease and experience less academic success. For many, though, it just means growing up with a marginal or strained relationship with their fathers.

The father of Anita Fields, a 38-year-old married mother who has two sons, spent most of Anita's childhood in prison. As Anita reflected on this, she described it this way:

> When I was growing up, my father was incarcerated on and off, since the time I was five. He then stayed in for 22 years [got out] and then he went back in. By the time my boys were born, he was locked up again. Mostly for drug

trafficking. He came out this last time in about 2012 and has done very well. He works, he's trying to keep up with his wife. I think he married her because it looked good on the books.

Anita loved her father and visited him over the years of his incarceration. She said she always felt like "daddy's little girl," and relished his recent complement that she was a good mother. "He told me he was proud of me, that I was a good mother. I always thought I was, but it was like with his assurance I never questioned it again. I feel like our fathers give us our identities."

The impact of having a mother incarcerated has received less attention, but in many cases it means that children are placed in foster care. The 30 percent increase in foster care between 1985 and 2000 was directly related to escalating rates of female incarceration. The Adoption and Safe Families Act 1997 mandated terminating the legal custody rights of parents whose children have been in foster care for 15 of the previous 22 months (Comfort, 2008). Thus, maternal incarceration and being in foster care have important implications for transmitting racial inequalities and poor life chances across generations, as both lead to adverse childhood outcomes. Anita's father, in fact, was the victim of a rough childhood that included the early deaths of family members and living with a grandmother who seemed to take in more foster children than she could manage:

> [My father's] parents died when he was young—his father was murdered when he was two years old. His brother died when he was five, and his mother died when he was nine. So there was just a lot of loss in his life, and he just didn't make good choices. He had a hard life, lived with his grandmother, in a bad part of town. She had a lot of foster children—about 60 over the years—and most of them did not do well. My dad didn't do well; he always had some kind of hustle going on.

Life after prison

The mass incarceration of the American population has now become a topic of a great deal of popular and scholarly attention. By 2004 there were six times more prison inmates and ex-inmates than in the 1970s, despite the fact that the crime rate was falling (Massoglia, 2008a,

2008b). Although the US has only 6 percent of the world's population, it has 25 percent of the world's prisoners. The racially based policies that have made young African-American men the primary targets of this incarceration have also been widely criticized. Black men were and still are six times more likely to be imprisoned than white men (Martin et al, 2015). Much of that incarceration is the result of the "war on drugs" and disproportionate sentencing for those found guilty of trafficking crack (rather than powder) cocaine.

The Department of Justice has passed policies aimed at narrowing the racial gap in penalties for drug use and trafficking, and initiated a process of releasing thousands of nonviolent prisoners each years. This has led to a growing "felon class" composed of millions of former felons who have re-entered society, most with no clear plan for building a new life (Uggen et al, 2006). Many lack job skills and had no strong connection to the labor market before incarceration, and in some cases did not have mainstream family roles (Western et al, 2015). Prison time has now become more about retribution than rehabilitation, and many leave prison without accomplishing anything positive, such as alcohol or drug treatment, work skills, or therapy. In many cases they are given a few dollars and a bus ticket, which they often use to return to the same troubled community they left. The probability of successfully integrating into mainstream society has declined over the years. In 1984, 70 percent of parolees completed their sentence without being re-arrested and gained their freedom, compared to 44 percent in 1996 and 33 percent in 2013 (Coates, 2015).

The process of being released after years of incarceration is stressful and can adversely affect the health of felons. People with a history of incarceration have high rates of infectious diseases and other chronic illnesses (Massoglia, 2008a, 2008b), and the risk of death for ex-convicts increases during their first few weeks out of prison (Wildeman, 2010; Wildeman and Western, 2010). Having been incarcerated is associated with mood and bipolar disorders and simply feeling "down," all of which relate to substance abuse and impulse control disorders (Schnittker et al, 2012). Older inmates and those with histories of mental illness or drug addiction are most likely to have difficulties reintegrating and to end up feeling socially isolated.

Being known as an "ex-con" comes with stigma and a loss of status, and often a cloud of suspicion where former inmates must continually prove their trustworthiness. Many also often find themselves members of a permanent underclass, as many are denied the right to vote or apply for public assistance. Laws in 30 states deny convicted felons on probation or parole the right to vote, and in two states they lose the right to vote for life—laws that have disenfranchised 13 percent of black men (Britton, 2011). In addition, welfare reform policies have placed a lifetime ban on public assistance for those convicted of drug felonies, a ban that especially affects low-income women and their children. Economic and material hardship is common among those released from prison, but many have few resources beyond the family. Many ex-convicts end up homeless. In Los Angeles and San Francisco, for example, between 30-50 percent of parolees are homeless (Coates, 2015).

Those who are paroled to complete their prison time under state or federal supervision often live in "mobile penitentiaries," since their homes and vehicles are targets of surveillance and can be searched at any time (Comfort et al, 2005). They are also subject to numerous conditions of parole, such as maintaining employment, having suitable living arrangements, and reporting regularly to parole officers. As an example, Megan Comfort shared the story of LaShawn and her partner, Darrell, who was paroled from prison after serving two years because he was a "model prisoner." Darrell returned to his family, got a job, and was doing so well that his parole officer allowed him to do his monthly paperwork at home instead of visiting the office. Darrell and LaShawn took their son to Disneyland for his birthday—a trip Darrell said was approved by his parole officer—but on return he was arrested and returned to prison for leaving the state, a devastating loss for LaShawn and her son:

> Here you take this man, the breadwinner, from the family. Okay, you cause a triple effect: you got another man in jail. You got a single parent now. You got a child without a father ... to me, they're not tryin' to help the problem taking' all our black men away and lockin' 'em up. (Comfort, 2008: 149)

Having been incarcerated undermines the two most health-producing activities in life—being employed and able to earn a living and being married and having strong family connections. Felons who manage to get a job earn considerably less than others; Wildeman and Western (2010) have argued that having been incarcerated reduces a man's earnings by up to 30 percent. Young black men are unlikely to be in a marital relationship, but those who are face a higher risk of divorce or separation during or after incarceration. Comfort (2008) has argued that during incarceration many couples create "romantic scripts" about what their lives will be like once they are back together that are difficult to achieve after the prisoner is released. Nevertheless, women—girlfriends, mothers, wives, daughters—are an important resource for released felons, especially in the early stages of reintegration. But incarceration often weakened or strained those relationships. Anita, mentioned earlier, felt she had a good relationship with her father during his incarceration, although it took a lot of time and money to stay connected. Still, when her father needed to live with her for a while on his release, she had to decline, saying, "I have two sons, and I can't have him around them. My dad, I love him, he's wonderful, but sometimes I have to say no."

Conclusion

Examining the impact of incarceration on black families and communities, Ta-Nehisi Coates concluded that:

> Peril is generational for black people in America—and incarceration is our current mechanism for ensuring the peril continues. Incarceration pushes you out of the job market. Incarceration disqualifies you from feeding your family with food stamps. Incarceration allows for housing discrimination based on a criminal-background check. Incarceration increases your risk of homelessness. Incarceration increases your risk of being incarcerated again. (Coates, 2015)

The economic decline that began in the 1970s and the epidemic of drugs and violence that ensued have had a devastating impact on black relationships and families, but none as devastating as the literally millions of Africans Americans who have been imprisoned. There is no doubt that incarceration was the right response to many of the crimes that were committed, yet the incarceration of black people for nonviolent offenses has reached an historic level. It has increased fatherlessness among black children, diminished the resources of low-income and poor families, fostered the spread of sickness and diseases, and left millions of kin and friends experiencing chronic stress over the welfare of their incarcerated loved ones.

SIX

Love, sexuality, and (non)marriage

Brownfield Copeland, a fictionalized character in *The third life of Grange Copeland*, is the son of black sharecroppers who is left mostly unattended by his parents, at least until he starts picking cotton at the age of six. His family lives in dire poverty in a two-room Georgia shack, where Brownfield watches his father "freeze up" with fear and humbleness when the white landowners come around. Outside their presence, however, he is a binge-drinking, womanizing, patriarchal tyrant who routinely beats his wife and berates her for not "selling herself" to help them escape poverty. After his father abandons the family and his mother commits suicide, Brownfield ventures North in search of work, where he falls deeply in love with and marries Mem, a school teacher. Brownfield wants the family life he never had, but his love turns to hatred and hostility when he is unable to provide for his family, and the fact that Mem can do so only intensifies his sense of failure. Increasingly humiliated, he convinces Mem to return to the South where he can find work as a sharecropper, just until something better comes long. Several years and three children later, however, he is still dragging his family from one sharecropping job to the next, falling deeper into hopelessness and poverty. Even worse, he has turned into the man he once despised—a womanizing, alcohol drinking husband and father who savagely beats his wife and heaps emotional abuse on his children.

Alice Walker, who has never shied away from controversial topics, published this novel in 1970, a time when many scholars were busy highlighting the strengths of black families. There is, in fact, impressive evidence of the strength and resiliency that African-American families have shown over the course of history—loving each other, marrying, and effectively raising children despite formidable challenges. The other side of the story is that racial oppression and desperate poverty take a devastating toll on families and the ability of couples to sustain loving relationships. Walker explained that the novel was based on a true incident she witnessed growing up in Eatonville, Georgia, where domestic violence was rampant (Walker, 1970). Donna Franklin, in her historic overview of African-American families, found that rates of domestic violence escalated among the newly freed slaves, as black men sought to create the patriarchal families prescribed by mainstream society (Franklin, 1997). Domestic violence has historically been common among married couples, leading feminist scholars to note that it occurs in "every walk of life." That truth, however, may mask the fact that economic hardship, having to struggle to survive, and being unable to adhere to conventional family and gender norms heightens the risk of violence. For many African Americans, those challenges are rooted in racial exclusion and racialized gendered stereotypes that can have a corrosive effect of relationships. This is the root of the "love and trouble" tradition between black men and women (Collins, 2004).

The health benefits of being loved and supported and having satisfying intimate partnerships and marriages have now been widely documented. On the other hand, being lonely, socially isolated, and in conflictual or exploitative social relationships takes a toll of the health of people of all ages. This chapter examines the consequences of love, sexuality, and marriage on the health and wellbeing of African Americans, specifically looking at how gender, racial, and class inequalities matter. Love and marriage are not inherently problematic for African Americans: one does not have to search hard to find successful black marriages or couples in committed relationships. Still, structural inequalities and gendered racism pose significant challenges to creating loving relationships, as evident in the low rates of marriage and high rates of divorce among African Americans. The impact of these inequalities on relationships undermines black health.

Love in a gender perspective

In the aftermath of the tumultuous civil rights and gender revolutions of the 1980s, African Americans' intimate relationships moved from the margins of scholarly attention to the center. Prior research had focused on black single mothers and the general resiliency (or lack thereof) of black families, but African Americans had been mostly excluded from studies focusing on dating, partnering, and marriage. In recent years this has changed, and even what was once seen hidden as "dirty laundry" has now emerged as a topic of open discussion—the difficulties black men and women have in forming loving and lasting relationships. Patricia Hill Collins described it as the "love and trouble" tradition, rooted in a history of racial, sexual, and gender oppression. The "love" aspect of that tradition is seen in the fact that the majority of African Americans partner, fall in love with and marry other black people, often forming relationships that last a lifetime. But the "trouble" black couples encounter in negotiating successful relationships goes beyond that found among most couples, as it unfolds in the context of the historic negation of and disregard for the lives, families, and marriages of black people. Many black people have found it difficult to abide by conventional gender and family ideologies and, more importantly, have been maligned and stigmatized for their inability to do so. Black men are characterized as sexually irresponsible and economic failures, and black women have been victimized by an array of demeaning stereotypes blaming them for emasculating men, dismissing the importance of husbands and fathers, and opting to depend on the government rather than a husband for economic support. Moreover, black women are seen as not meeting culturally valued norms of femininity and attractiveness.

These racialized gender stereotypes have cast a long shadow over black relationships; indeed, black people who are far removed from the academy and have never heard of the Moynihan Report often bemoan the "gender disorder" among African Americans, the belief that men are unable or unwilling to support their families and are too quick to abandon them, and that women are domineering and controlling. Gender traditionalism is common in the attitudes of African Americans, often based on their religious beliefs or efforts to achieve respectability in the dominant society. Tensions over gender ideologies help predict lower levels of love among black married men and higher rates of marital discord and divorce (Stanik et al, 2013).

The gender dilemma of African-American men and women took an interesting turn during the civil rights era, especially with the burgeoning of feminism during the 1970s. Black women went from being demeaned as "matriarchs"—at least among most scholars—to being seen as exemplars of the strength and independence that all women should strive for. The historic experiences of African-American women, such as managing to combine labor market work with caring for their families—often without the support of a male partner— offered a substantial challenge to essentialist notions of womanhood. To some extent, black womanhood was valorized; for example, black women have been heralded as pioneers in the evolution of dual-income families and the egalitarian gender norms that have now become widely accepted (Landry, 2000).

Notions of black masculinity did not fare nearly as well. On the one hand, historians mustered some evidence that challenged the idea that enslaved black men were marginal members of families, such as noting that they contributed to providing for their families (Gutman, 1976). The 1970s also saw a new assertion of black masculinity in the broader culture, such as movies starring invincible black heroes (for example, *Shaft*) and a highly masculinized black power movement. But these efforts to redeem black masculinity were soon overshadowed by their growing rates of unemployment, homicide, and incarceration, which led to a counter-narrative that described black men as part of the "underclass" or a "vanishing species."

Economic marginalization and negative racialized gender stereotypes still leave many African-American men and women on the sidelines when it comes to enduring, romantic relationships, sometimes blaming each other for failing to meet societal norms and for their relationship difficulties. The status gap between them poses further challenges: black women earn less than black men, but they are more likely to have a college education and especially an advanced degree, and this affects their values and relationship choices. In a national study of African-American women's experiences, Charisse Jones and Kumea Shorter-Gooden highlight some of the difficulties women have when they are seen as more ambitious than their male counterparts. One woman, for example, noted that she had been successful in everything she had endeavored to do—except have a romantic relationship with a black man:

> I have always, always had a problem with black men. I used to think it was something wrong with me, but now I know it's because I was ambitious at a very early age, and I had goals. I don't think I was that smart. I just have mother wit. I must accomplish something every year in my life. Men always had problems with me. I was bossy, I was too much. (Jones and Shorter-Gooden, 2003: 219)

Although black women have a status advantage, men still have more power when it comes to choosing whom to date and marry. Not all women are eager to marry and most are pretty selective about who to marry, but as a rule they are more marriage-minded than men and more interested in being in a stable, committed relationship. But black women face a tight marriage market because of the skewed gender ratio, or the fact that they outnumber black men.

Movies such as *Waiting to exhale* and *The brothers* that depict black women as eagerly pursuing intimacy and marriage and black men as reluctant to take the plunge are popular because they resonate with the experiences of so many middle-class African Americans. The difficulties have also been the topic of a few academic studies. Examining dating and sexual relationships among students at an elite university, one study found that black females, more than any other race/gender group, expressed the strongest desire for someone to date. As one black student said, "There are some people dating within the black community, it's just that guys aren't willing to do it more than once … with one female" (quoted in McClintock, 2010). African-American females in this study felt they simply did not have the same opportunities to date as black men, especially in the area of interracial dating. Although some black women did get involved in interracial "hookups," their nonblack male partners often wanted to keep the relationship a secret.

Law professor Ralph Richard Banks' longstanding interest in race and marriage led him to conduct research on the marriage decline among middle-class black people. He explored theories generally used to explain it, for example, the legacy of slavery, black cultural traditions, generous welfare policies, and the shortage of black marriageable men. Banks found some support for each theory, but the most compelling evidence was for the shortage of black marriageable men. But there was more to the story: black men exploited the abundance of African-American women by foregoing marriage and having concurrent sexual relationships. One result is loneliness and depression among many black women, emotional states which have been associated with elevated blood pressure and poor cardiovascular health (Carr and Springer, 2010) as well as poor self- esteem and depression (Jones and Shorter-Gooden, 2003).

In *Inequalities in love*, Averil Clarke also interviewed middle-class black women about their search for intimacy and documented the impact of racial and gender inequalities in access to love. Her central argument is that college-educated black women are deprived and maligned in sexual and reproductive relations, leading to singleness, unrequited love and, for many, betraying their own moral standards in order to find a man (Clarke, 2011). Gender and cultural traditions give men the power to select partners and determine who is attractive and eligible for monogamous love, long-term relationships, or marriage. Most of the college-educated black women Clarke interviewed wanted to be in a loving and intimate relationship, but they were also striving to create identities and lives that contradicted racialized gender stereotypes that cast them as sexually immoral or as single mothers. This left them even more vulnerable in their relationships. For example, many did not plan to have casual or nonmarital sex but ended up doing so, exposing themselves to the risks of unwanted pregnancy and sexually transmitted diseases, not to mention the risk of just feeling used. Black women have a lower likelihood of ever marrying and as a group spend fewer of their reproductive years in marriage. So, for those interested in becoming mothers—and most were—nonmarital fertility was the only option.

Black sexuality

Black sexuality has often been more a topic of speculation and derision than scientific study. In *Exploring black sexuality*, Robert Staples (2006) sought to advance the scholarly discourse on the topic in a book that explored almost every aspect of black sexuality, from sexual norms in pre-colonial Africa through slavery and modern times. He argued that many African nations had strict sexual rules, but they differed from European or Christian ideals, and led to Africans being seen as "sexual savages." This characterization served colonizers and slave traders well, as it enabled them to exploit African sexuality for personal and economic gain. Declaring that black people were lacking any sense of sexual morality made it possible for colonists to deny Africans control over their own bodies and to propagate demeaning sexual stereotypes and practices. Black women were characterized as sexually immoral "jezebels" and black men as "bucks," and rape, slave breeding, and nonmarital sex were normative. Racialized notions of sexuality remain common and are key to the maintenance of racism. As Collins has noted: "Black people carry the stigma of promiscuity or excessive or unrestrained heterosexual desire. This is the sexual deviancy that has both been assigned to Black people and been used to construct racism" (Collins, 2004: 97).

Staples has contended that these experiences and stereotypes are the basis for more liberal sexual attitudes and practices among African Americans, although there were other influences, such as the fact that their sexual experiences were not motivated by material rewards. African Americans are the "trailblazers for the sexual freedom that most Americans today embrace," wrote Staples. But he supported that thesis by noting that sexuality is a dominant theme in black literature, music, and comedy and highlighting the sexual exploits of black celebrities, pimps, and prostitutes—despite the fact that these sexual bahaviors do not reflect the sexual values of most black Americans. Despite this greater liberalism, Staples maintained that black women are less interested in sex than white women, and that black people have fewer enjoyable sexual experiences due to their high rates of poor health, low self-esteem, obesity, and substance abuse. Sex, however, has often been a haven from racial oppression, an observation Staples shares with other scholars. In one study, for example, one black woman suggested that sexual encounters were a way of addressing feelings of inferiority and of not being loved:

> Sexuality for us [Blacks] has become a sedative … with the stresses of our lives and some of the things we deal with…. I see people who struggle with self-esteem issues, who struggle economically, who have so many disparities … that to have a moment where you feel good, to have a moment when you feel loved, is something that many people are seeking after. (quoted in Barnes, 2013: 117-18)

Sex is rarely exclusively about love or sexual desire, but has the potential for being more exploitative in the context of racial, gender, and class inequalities. Research shows that the onset of sexuality is earlier for African Americans than for Whites, but the difference is related to their economic resources, adult role models, and religious beliefs (Brewster, 1994). One study found that neighborhood disadvantage was a major reason that African-American adolescents have more favorable attitudes towards sexual activity and nonmarital childbearing, although diminished social control by parents and individual factors also mattered (Browning et al, 2008). Substance abuse and depression are also factors that explain the sexual behaviors of many adolescents (Jackson et al, 2015). Although there are legitimate reasons to be concerned about the sexual behaviors of adolescents, racial comparisons run the risk of reinforcing notions of black sexual immorality. Racial differences in sexuality may be less relevant today, since the majority of people—95 percent—engage in sex prior to marriage (Cohen, 2015) and on average, females are sexually active for 10 years before getting married (Paquette, 2015).

Sexual relationships remain highly gendered, and the double standard of sexuality common. Women are more likely to want sexuality to unfold in or lead to a relationship. Younger and low-income black females are often caught in the bind of being sexually available but selective and being judged by their appearances. As one young single mother said:

> Men are interested in what's untouched, in what's pure. They're not interested in a woman with a baby.... Most men like women with the perfect measurements, no children, no sex or they had a little sex, but you don't know a lot about sex. You don't have to have a mind or brain, you can be dumb, but you have the looks, the body. (quoted in Hutchinson, 1999: 77)

Same-sex relationships and HIV/AIDS

Attitudes about same-sex relationships have changed significantly in the US during the past few decades, with the majority of people now supporting gay and lesbian rights. African Americans, however, are less accepting of same-sex relationships than white Americans, arguably because they link it with a longstanding theme of black sexual deviance. Jenkins has argued that Blacks' aversion to homosexuality is the result of efforts to be seen as conforming to conventional sexual norms, thus avoiding the double vulnerability of racial and sexual deviance (Jenkins, 2007). Many people equate being authentically black with heterosexism and view male homosexuality as the result of white oppression or white efforts at black genocide (Collins 2004), attitudes which also marginalize people in same-sex relationships. Despite these concerns, African Americans appear more likely to identify as gay, bisexual, lesbian, or transgender than other racial groups (Coles, 2016).

The extent that bisexual or closeted gay black men have sex with or maintain their primary relationship with women has been a topic of recent discussion, but often within a negative framework that describes them as being on the "down low." These men are seen as deceitful manipulators who unwittingly and/or uncaringly expose their partners to sexually transmitted diseases, especially HIV/AIDS. Some scholars, however, have taken exception to the "down low" concept, especially the notion that it is an exclusively black phenomenon, that the women involved are the innocent victims of it, and that it has contributed substantially to the HIV/AIDS epidemic among African Americans (Robinson, 2009). One survey of 21 US cities where black men have sex with other men found that 21 percent of them had also had a female sex partner in the past year. Some women were unaware of this and heartbroken to discover their partner's sexuality infidelity, but others were not and did not end the relationship. In at least a few cases, the women felt closer to their partners after they had learned of the relationship. As one 51-year-old woman said:

> He told me that he's a man, he's a full man, but he was in prison for 15 years, and he missed being with a woman, and things just happened. And he's not proud of it, but they happened and they're in the past, so I let them stay in the past. I was like, 'my God, you're so manly.' But I didn't hold it against him. People make mistakes.

While sexual orientation remains a hot issue in black communities, there is little evidence that gay and bisexual men are contributing significantly to the spread of HIV/AIDS. Still, STDs are extremely high among African Americans, especially teenagers and young adults; for example, nearly half of all newly reported cases are found in black females between the ages of 15 and 24 (Pflieger et al, 2013). Assortive mating—or partnering with those within your own racial groups—and having concurrent sexual partners or a short duration between sexual partners are major factors in the prevalence of HIV/AIDS and other STDs in black communities (Pflieger et al, 2013).

Unwanted pregnancy and childbirth

One recent study of sexuality among single women who were not planning to get pregnant found that those who were poor were five times more likely than those who were affluent to have an unintended pregnancy. Although there were no differences in sexual promiscuity, access to reliable birth control did vary: poor women had less access to sex education and contraceptives and were less likely to abort an unwanted pregnancy (Paquette, 2015).

Other adverse consequences of sexuality fall disproportionately to the poor and African Americans. Nearly half of all pregnancies in the US are unplanned, unwanted, or mistimed, but the prevalence of such pregnancies is greater among those who are young, unmarried, poor, African American, and those who are the least able to care for their children (Guzzo and Hayford, 2014). Those who are young and black also have more adverse birth outcomes, such as low-weight infants. Pregnancy and childbearing before the age of 20 is associated with inadequate prenatal care and a negative impact on health over the life span: it increases the risks of early death and, among those who reach midlife, is correlated with higher rates of cancer, heart disease, and lung disease (Henretta, 2007). Those who have multiple children and poor prenatal and infant nutrition are more likely to have diabetes in adulthood (Henretta, 2007).

Decline of marriage

People today are much less likely to get or stay married than they were in past, but the decline in marriage among African Americans has been sharper than that for other racial groups. The average age of first marriage is later today than in the past—29 for men and 27 for women. Black women have an even later age of first marriage—30.4 years old—and are less likely to marry at all. Today, about 80 percent of people have married at least once by the age of 50, but this represents a sharp decline in marriage compared to the 1970s (Cohen, 2015). At the current rate, only about 61% of black women will marry. The number of years that people between the ages of 18 and 55 spend married has declined—from 29 years in 1960 to 19 in 2010 (Cohen, 2015).

In *Marriage-go-round*, Andrew J. Cherlin (2009) has argued that marriage as a cultural ideal is stronger in the US than in comparable Western countries, a fact that stands in sharp contrast to our higher divorce rate. This contradiction is explained by two important American values—religion and individuality. The US remains one of the most religious nations in the Western world, as measured by attendance at worship services and professions of belief in God. As a result, many conservative religionists and politicians promote marriage, and even see it as the only legitimate context for having sex and children. Thus, marriage has remained a major cultural value, "the most prestigious way to live your life," and a symbol of success. On the other hand, individualism promotes the importance of freedom, personal growth, and the right to happiness, so people simply do not feel obliged to stay in marriages unless they support those values. In the past, leaving unsatisfying marital unions may have been untenable, but the entry of women into the labor market, the liberalization of sexual norms, and the growing diversity of family structures have made it more acceptable.

The question then becomes, who marries, and why? People who have more class resources, especially a college education, are more likely to marry and stay married, and they have more to gain by doing so—more wealth, social respectability, and stability. College-educated people marry at a later age and so are likely to be better prepared emotionally and financially for marital success (Cherlin, 2013). Lower- and working-class people also marry, especially those who are religious, but they have more trouble acquiring the resources they need to sustain the marriage and higher rates of divorce. In recent decades there has been a trend for low-income women of all races, including those who are single mothers, to pass on the opportunity to marry. Many hold marriage in high esteem, as the most respectable way to form a family, but they are not confident that they have the resources to marry. Those resources go beyond jobs and money and include finding men they can trust, men who are not abusive, and men who will remain sexually faithful to them (Edin and Kefalas, 2011).

Social class intersects with the racial and/or cultural traditions of African Americans in shaping their marriage patterns. Black people are as likely as others to express strong attitudinal support for marriage, but they are the least likely to marry. Marriage has never been as strongly institutionalized among black people, arguably due to African traditions that prioritized blood over marital ties, but also because they were not allowed to enter legal marriage contracts during slavery. While there is evidence that African Americans sought to legalize their unions after slavery ended, there was also a strong nonmarital ethos that prevailed, especially among black women, who were used to being single mothers and gained little by marrying (Hill, 2005, 2006).

The gender division of labor upheld in a traditional marriage contract was also less applicable to African Americans, especially its stipulations about exclusive sexual and property rights and transfers of wealth. Still, by the 1950s, African Americans were as likely as Whites to marry (Koball, 1998), but significantly less likely to be able to sustain those marriages. The rate of divorce among African Americans has historically been and remains twice that of Whites (Franklin, 2000; Coles, 2016). Today, single motherhood is common in black communities (and increasingly elsewhere), and no one is surprised when a pregnant woman decides not to marry.

Laura Times was 23 when she got pregnant, and pointed out: "I wasn't ready and didn't plan it. I *did not* plan it!" She continued to work, as did her boyfriend, who held two jobs:

> We both stayed with my parents. He asked me to marry him but I said just because I'm pregnant doesn't mean we need to get married. You actually have to love one another and lead up to that. I knew he wasn't ready, so I said no. It crushed his heart. But I didn't want to get married

just because I was pregnant, because that doesn't mean a marriage will work.

The relationship ended a couple of years later, and Laura went on to have a second child, fathered by another man, but she has never married. She has a long employment history, mostly working for an insurance company, and sees being a single mother as normal. "Shotgun weddings"—or marriages that are inspired by pregnancy—are pretty much a thing of the past.

Family background and religion are important factors in who decides to marry, although they do not always spare couples from divorce. For example, Brenda Lancaster is a 62-year-old happily married mother of two adult sons. She grew up in a rural area in a family composed of both parents and six children and had what she described as "perfect childhood" of working on the farm, playing outside, and hunting and fishing. Brenda had a stay-at-home mother, at least for most of her childhood, and a father who worked for more than 30 years as an auto mechanic before becoming a full-time farmer. In the mid-1970s she graduated from high school and went to college, but she returned home after one semester because there was so much racial unrest on campus ("the Black Panthers basically took over the dorms!"). Someone on campus was shot and killed, and her protective father decided that going back to college was too dangerous.

Brenda moved back home, enrolled at a junior college, and was introduced by a friend to the man who became her first husband—they were both in the church choir. Because of their religious beliefs, they did not even consider having sex before marriage, and in order to plan her pregnancies, she started birth control before marrying. Brenda was shocked when her parents divorced after nearly 40 years of marriage, but she later decided to end her own marriage.

Research by A. Perry found that family structure and religion shaped the marriage attitudes of young African-American men, along with how they scored on a fear of intimacy survey (Perry, 2013). For many black men, living in two-parent families and witnessing marital stability among at least some of those around them were important factors in shaping their marriage attitudes. One 22-year-old man, who was considering proposing to his girlfriend, pointed to the married couples in his own family and wished stable marriages were more the norm these days:

It's like ... my grandparents have been together before, like since before I could remember. I have an auntie and uncle that have been together since the sixth grade. You know, and I'm like I want that. But when there is a certain standard ... so entrenched in your family that you don't know any other way, then that's just how it is.

Although growing up in a stable family of origin can foster pro-marriage attitudes among young men, other family and developmental factors may have the opposite influence. At a time when most young men are moving into steady relationships based on sexual fidelity and commitment, African-American men often still have multiple sexual partners and high levels of conflictual, unsatisfying relationships. Poverty, racial stereotypes, and deprivation shape their relationship experiences, but so does growing up in families with less stringent behavioral expectations, less supervision, and having higher rates of harsh parenting (Kogan et al, 2016).

Marriage and health

Although marriage is ideally about love and creating a satisfying family, many conservative policy-makers and scholars have come to champion the value of marriage in solving the problems of poverty, welfare dependency, and poor childhood outcomes. Marriage does not pull all families out of poverty or eliminate the risk of economic hardship, but it does diminish the odds. Recent data show that 25 percent of families composed of married parents and children earn less than $38,000 a year (150 percent of the poverty guideline for a family of four), compared to 60 percent of single-parent families. But beyond earnings, many have pointed to the health benefits of marriage (Carr and Springer, 2010). The link between health and marriage has been documented for a least a century, with studies finding that married people have lower rates of death than unmarried people, a life span advantage that still exists. Married couples, a more recent study found, tend to monitor each other's health behaviors, such as sleeping, eating, and alcohol consumption, help spouses detect health problems, and encourage them to visit doctors (Miller et al, 2013). Marriage also provides the social support that protects people against the harmful effects of stress, thus enhancing physical and psychological wellbeing.

In a summary of research done in recent decades, Parker-Pope found that married people, compared to those who are unmarried, have lower rates of dementia, surgery, heart attacks, cancer, and violent death (Parker-Pope, 2010). These marital benefits are related to the economic advantages of married-couple families, as most have two wage earners, but also to the fact that marriage is the most positively sanctioned living arrangement, and an indicator of love and stability. Being married is a source of status: it was found to boost the self-esteem of low-income Black women as much as money did for their unmarried and more affluent counterparts (Mandara et al, 2008).

Although the link between marriage and health has been strongly supported, more research needs to be done on how that health advantage varies based on social class, race, and other aspects of married life. There is some evidence that African Americans do not reap the same level of health or wealth benefits from marriage as Whites, since those benefits are related to being in happy and supportive marriages. Several factors predict lower marital satisfaction among African Americans and higher rates of divorce. Entering a marriage with children increases the likelihood of divorce: more than half of all African Americans already have children before they marry and, of those who do, half have children by more than one partner (Stanik et al, 2013). Even among low-income couples, Blacks enter marriage with fewer economic resources: they have less education and higher rates of unemployment at the time of marriage (Jackson et al, 2014).

The support married couples receive from family members and friends also influences their success. Extended black kin networks can work against marital happiness, as they can undermine the primacy of the marriage relationship. One study found that wives in kin-centered units are less likely to discuss their problems with their husbands and more likely to experience marital dissatisfaction (Milardo and Graham, 2000). Overall, African-American couples receive less family support than their white counterparts, and black wives are especially likely to report a lack of emotional support (Jackson et al, 2014). Black couples in this study had fewer duocentric networks—people who appeared in both spouse's social networks—and were less likely to feel close to their partner's family.

Gender attitudes and practices also affect levels of marital satisfaction. Although some early research found that black couples have relatively egalitarian relationships, studies comparing them with other racial groups have not necessarily confirmed this. Black husbands often do more around the house than white husbands, but they do not share equally (John and Shelton, 1997), and black couples experience more conflict over work–family responsibilities than white couples, especially if the wife has a career (Bridges and Orza, 1996). Among newlywed black couples, both husbands and wives report lower marital quality when the husband has a traditional gender ideology (Stanik et al, 2013).

Gender attitudes are likely implicated in the fact that, even when social class and income are controlled for, African Americans experience more husband-to-wife violence than Hispanics or Whites (McLoyd et al, 2000). The prospect of intimate partner violence is higher in unhappy and conflictual marriages, and the fear of battering is one reason that low-income women are reluctant to marry. In many urban areas, between 5 to 38 percent of all young mothers experience interpersonal violence either during or after their pregnancies (Mitchell et al, 2010). Mitchell found that young black mothers, on average, had experienced five episodes of violence—ranging from being slapped or hit (62 percent) to being shot (6 percent)—and had witnessed more than 26 episodes of violence. One low-income black mother interviewed by Edin described the advantage of being single as "not living with someone there to abuse you. I'm not sacred anymore. I'm scared for my bills and I'm scared of if I get sick, what's going to happen to my kids, but I'm not afraid for my life" (quoted in Edin, 2000).

The majority of studies find that African Americans are not as happily married as Whites (McLoyd et al, 2000; Stanik and Bryant, 2012), and this is especially the case for black women who have a higher status than their partner (LaPierre and Hill, 2013). Children living in families where marital conflict is high have more psychological distress and more externalizing behaviors (McLoyd et al, 2000). Thus, while good marriages very likely enhance the health and wealth of both spouses, marriages that are unhappy and stress-filled may have the opposite impact, as poor relationships or those that deteriorate over time lead to worsening health (Barr et al, 2013).

Conclusion

Married life remains highly appealing for the majority of Americans, most of whom plan to marry. In many ways marriage is the penultimate intimate relationship, ideally a partnership where love, sexuality, and social support are combined in a committed union. Further research, however, is needed to explore how its presumed health and wealth benefits are affected by social class, racial, and gender inequalities. Economic transitions and changing gender and sexual norms have also made the path from courtship to marriage bumpier for all couples, intensifying relationship strains that have always been common among African Americans. In this chapter, I have suggested that the adverse health consequences of these relationships fall primarily to women in the form of sexually transmitted diseases, unplanned and unwanted pregnancies, and psychological and emotional distress. More research clearly needs to be done to explore how relationship issues affect the health of black men and same-sex couples. It is evident, however, that they affect the quality of life for children, which is the topic of the final chapter.

SEVEN

Children's health

Families have changed dramatically over the past few decades with the entry of more women into the labor market, more people delaying or foregoing marriage, more nonmarital cohabitation, more single parents, an increasing number of stepfamilies, and the legalization of same-sex marriage. Only a minority of US families conforms to what was once thought of as the traditional family—a married, heterosexual couple with dependent children living together in a breadwinner-homemaker family. Most have come to accept that family changes are inevitable and the result of a changing economy, greater individual freedom, and growing support for gender and sexual equality. Yet, from a political and personal standpoint, family changes spark concern and controversy. The most compelling reason is that families have at least two important responsibilities, namely, reproducing and socializing children. For many, the proliferation of new family forms not only challenges longstanding and often religiously sanctioned notions about the sanctity of marriage, but they pose a threat to the welfare of children. How do children fare living with unmarried or cohabitating parents, in stepfamilies, or with parents of the same sex? Do these families have an adverse effect on children? Are these families and children more likely to require state aid or intervention?

The latter part of the 20th century witnessed tense debates over the balance between public and private responsibility for children. A significant majority of people believe that parents should be responsible for providing economically for their children, but are divided on why they may not be able to do so and how the state should respond when they cannot. Progressives tend to believe that family changes are fueled by a changing economy, which has made it more difficult for people to earn livable wages, and that we should recognize and support the legitimacy of diverse families. Most support greater public investments to ensure the welfare of children. Conservatives lean towards framing the issue as a decline in cultural values, and see the solution as curtailing welfare programs. Although welfare policies to aid children in poor families were implemented in the 1930s and extended in the 1960s, they often remain highly contested. This is especially the case when it comes to providing welfare to poor never-married single-mother families which, some conservatives have argued, is the major social problem facing the US and a key factor in the perpetuation of poverty (Murray, 1984). Overall, single-mother families (30.6 percent) are nearly five times more likely than married-couple families (5.8 percent) to live in poverty. Single-mother families are also much more likely to be living in near-poverty or low-income households.

This chapter examines the health of African-American children in the context of families and the broader community. I first look at how parents describe their children's health and the health socialization of their children, or what they teach them about staying healthy. I devote attention to the sexual socialization parents are providing for their children, an especially relevant aspect of health socialization for black children given their rates of unplanned pregnancy and sexually transmitted diseases (STDs). The health socialization provided by parents is influenced by their social class position and what they are actually able to provide for their children, along with the broader social context of neighborhoods and schools. For many African-American children, the latter are high-risk environments and, along with race and class disadvantage, this complicates the ability of children to develop healthy identities and lifestyles. Overall, African-American children experience many health challenges because they are subject to the same racial, class, and gender inequities as black adults.

Promoting health and health behaviors

In a sense, children have been the major beneficiaries of the epidemiological transition of better health and longer life spans, as rates of infant and childhood mortality have declined sharply in modern societies. Although the actual racial disparity did not change much over the course of the 20th century—it remains twice as high for Blacks as for Whites—the actual decline in infant and early childhood death has been dramatic for all racial groups. Most parents expect their children to survive and be healthy, and most of the parents I interviewed saw their children enjoying good health. For example, while only one or two parents described their own health as "excellent," many described their children's health that way. Sheryl Hadley, a 42-year-old single mother of two children, described her 13-year-old daughter this way:

> My daughter's health is excellent. She is very active and very intelligent—I know parents say that about their children, but she really is. She is in the 8th grade, and really not an athletic child but she's in dance class and she does hip-hop, so that's movement.... She wants to go to UCLA and be an obstetrician, or maybe a college in Texas or Florida.

Sheryl is a low-income mother who works at a Christian day care center. Like most parents she is proud of her two children and doing her best to be a good mother. She does not do anything explicitly to teach her daughter about staying healthy, but thinks they both benefit from the fact that she has given up red meat—once she was on her own, she discovered it was just too expensive.

Most parents saw their children as naturally healthy but usually had to think about what they actually did to help their children stay healthy. The most common responses to the question of what they were doing or teaching their children about good health were general dietary things, like making sure they ate fruit and vegetables and giving them vitamins. Some related the question to how they dealt with their child's sicknesses. Describing her 10-year-old son, Rosemary said:

> He doesn't have full-blown asthma but from time to time he gets the wheezing, little coughing and that's when he has to take the inhaler.... I guess as a mom you never really sleep straight through but it mostly hits him throughout the night.

Asthma is a common childhood health problem in the US, and is more common among Blacks than Whites. Nearly 21 percent of all black children have at one time in their life been diagnosed with having asthma, compared to 12 percent of white children (Warren et al, 2012).

Another childhood disorder that has become prevalent among children in the US is attention deficit hyperactivity disorder (ADHD). The children of a few mothers noted this health challenge, but saw it as manageable. The mother of an eight-year-old described her daughter as "shutting down around other children" and "reluctant to make friends." Still, she emphasized her positive attributes and the effective management of her ADHD:

> She's very creative and likes activities. Her life is busy—she's in dance classes. She was diagnosed with ADHD when she was five. Her teacher told us about it and gave her some tests. She has systems sound disorder—she constantly stutters, but it's part of her ADHD. She's on medication—a steroid. It's the third one she's been on, but this one is working.... She likes taking it, she says it helps her try her best.

Most frequently mentioned as a health issue was the early onset of obesity. Research has found that 13 percent of African-American children are overweight or obese, and that obesity is strongly related to family structure—those in low-income single-mother families have higher rates (Schmeer, 2012). Obesity among black children is more likely than among white children to be linked to diabetes mellitus, stroke, and high cholesterol (Outley, 2006). Several of the mothers I spoke with saw this as the major health issue with their children. Marsha Gray described the early maturation of her 12-year-old daughter, her daughter's discomfort with having big "boobs" at such an early age, and her pattern of sporadic dieting and dissatisfaction with her body:

> The thing that she struggles with is her weight—she has a tendency to eat or want to eat more than she needs to. If we get pizza, she'll put three pieces on her plate. She grew up a lot faster than other girls her age; she wears a size 40 bra, her cycle started early, when she was seven, and the doctor had her take depo shots [birth control] until she was nine.... She's not a kid that likes physical activity, like sports and things, so she doesn't get into any of that.

The health socialization provided by parents is often complemented by that offered by the health care system and in schools. Asked about her 12-year-old daughter's health behaviors, Jackie said:

> My 12-year-old is healthy. She doesn't drink pop—only water. Seldom does she eat candy. She loves vegetables. She is always asking 'is that healthy, Mom?' I think she gets it from school, but she's always interested in what's healthy. But she does like McChicken, but that is about the only thing she does that's not good for her health.

Lacy Edwards and her five-year-old son are learning health behaviors from a nutrition program she was referred to because her son is overweight and diabetes runs in the family. Her son enjoys the attention he receives from being in the nutrition program for children sponsored by the hospital and is already taking an active role in his health:

> He's healthy [but] they consider him obese so we're working on getting that taken care of. We go see a nutritionist and whatever they ask me to do I try to comply with, you know, like changing his eating habits and keeping him active. I'm a diabetic and his dad's side of the family has diabetes in the family as well, so its just one of those things. They say it's going to be natural for him to be a diabetic. He was a big baby when he was born, so he basically has been overweight all his life. Actually, he is really into changing his eating habits … so he's instructing me on what he needs me to buy him.

Some research has shown that children start to develop their health lifestyles early in life and that those lifestyles have long-term implications. Mollborn and associates, focusing on preschool children, found that they develop their own health lifestyles based on the health socialization of their parents and overall family context. They are taught or exposed to a number of factors that promote or impair their health, such as nutrition, sleeping patterns, and smoking (Mollborn et al, 2014). Over time, however, children transition from a received health lifestyle to an achieved health lifestyle, which is affected by the family and broader culture. For many children, for example, the media play a major role in their health behaviors. Research has found that children as young as two to six years old view about two hours of television each day, and those between the ages of six and eleven as much as 23 hours a week. A content analysis of advertisements on children's after-school television programs found that those more popular among black children—for example, shows featuring black children (*That's so Raven*) or aired on black television networks—were more likely to have advertisements that promoted poor eating behaviors (Outley, 2006).

Sexuality and sex education

The sexual socialization of children is an important part of childrearing, even more so for African Americans given their high rates early initiation into sex, STDs, and unintended pregnancy. The sexual norms and behaviors of Americans have shifted toward more liberal attitudes over the course of history. The historic ideal was that sex should occur only within marriage (an ideal that was widely violated), but most people today approve of sex between consenting adults. Beginning with those born in 1960, about 95 percent of Americans have sex before marriage, a trend fueled by access to birth control, delayed marriage, and greater independence from parents (Cohen, 2015). Although there is widespread acceptance of nonmarital sex, sex among teenagers remains controversial, even more so if they fail to use precautions against the adverse consequences of being sexually active.

The extent to which teenage sexuality leads to STDs, pregnancy, or childbirth is related to their exposure to sex education, access to birth control, and the general social context of their lives. Cohen (2015) has pointed out that teenagers in the US become sexually active around the same age as teens in comparable nations, but are more likely to get pregnant, contract diseases, and have babies because attitudes about sex are less open, as evidenced by debates over sex education. Many parents believe that teaching children about sexuality is their responsibility, as they are in the best position to know what to teach their children and when. Yet research has consistently shown that parents across races, social classes, and generations are notoriously ineffective when it comes to talking to their children about sex (Elliott, 2012).

The most frequent answer I received when I asked respondents what their own parents had taught them about sex was "nothing," or close to it. One respondent said: "My mother was very religious—that was my teaching, wait until you get married. That was pretty much it." Another said: "I think my mother didn't want me to learn about sex," explaining that when a sex education class was offered at her school, her mother did not give her permission to take it. Although she grew up in a middle-class family, she was pregnant by the age of 17 and did not see it as a problem as her older sister was a teenage mother:

> I was 17 when I got pregnant.... I didn't plan a pregnancy. My older sister had her first child at 13 and lived in and out of the house. I was following in her footsteps, wanting to do whatever she was doing, especially her and the baby getting attention.

Most parents, especially middle-class parents, are devastated when their teenage daughters get pregnant. It diminishes their own sense of respectability, compromises the futures of their children, and often leaves them obligated to help take care of a baby. Bethany's parents were very disappointed to learn she was pregnant and, although they had already experienced the pregnancy of her sister, refused to speak to Bethany for the first six or seven months of the pregnancy, which also meant that she did not get prenatal health care until late in the pregnancy.

Many people believe that sex education classes in school actually encourage teenagers to have sex, especially when those programs offer information about birth control. Welfare reform policies, despite embracing the explicit goal of reducing nonmarital childbirth, advocated teaching abstinence-only sex education. The federal government designated $50 million annually to states willing to provide matching grants to develop such classes, with the stipulation that two key principles be taught: the important social, psychological, and health gains that come from sexual abstinence, and that abstinence was the only sure way to avoid STDs and pregnancy. These programs are often intense—some require 50 hours of instruction and others meet every day of the school year—yet an evaluation of abstinence programs found no significant difference in rates of teenage sexuality between participants and nonparticipants (Trenholm et al, 2008). Still, as of 2013, about half of all states still required teaching abstinence as sex education, while no more than 17 required teaching contraception methods (Cohen, 2015).

Most of the parents I spoke with were not much better than schools when it came to teaching their children about sex. There is a tendency for every generation of parents to believe teenage sexuality is rampant or fear that their children will be exposed to it prematurely through the media or their peers, but they are reluctant to see their own children as potentially sexual beings. Bethany, who became a mother at age 17, plans to talk to her own daughter about sex when the times comes. But despite her experience, says she cannot imagine a circumstance under which she would help her get birth control before the age of 18:

> I haven't told her about sexuality; I'll tell her once she starts her period. I'll give her information about sex, that there's nothing wrong with it. I will tell her she needs to wait until she is married, but come to me if she wants to be sexually active before that. [*What if she comes to you at age 15 wanting birth control?*] I would probably try to play it cool and convince her that it's not her time; she should wait and focus on other things. I'd find her something else to do and get her mind off of it. I can't think of any circumstances under which I'd help her get birth control before she's 18.

Most of the parents I spoke to, even those with adolescent children, refused to consider that their children might be interested in sex. As one mother said of her 11-year-old son:

> It hasn't come to that right now. [*Would he be able to say what sex is?*] No, but we are getting closer.... We are not surrounding him with those ideas; even the TV is censored. I don't want to introduce him to that right now when we are trying to keep his mind focused on other things.... If a sexual scene comes up on TV—it's still a little gross to him. I want him talking to me, though, about sex and no one else.

For some parents, the question about sex education was taken to mean education about being inappropriately touched or, more commonly, about homosexuality. Mothers denied their preadolescent sons had any awareness of or interest in sex, and felt that they could protect them from learning about it. One mother, speaking of her 10-year-old, said:

> No, we haven't really talked about [sex]. We think he is not mature enough to handle that information yet ... he possesses a certain innocence. We do discuss things like marriage, couples, and homosexuality, what the Bible says about it. We discuss things like that but we don't discuss actual intercourse. We talked about protecting himself from other people or being careful about people who are approaching him in an inappropriate way.

More educated parents were more open to talking to their children about sex and, if they absolutely had to, helping them get birth control. Camille, a married mother of two, said of her children (ages 10 and 11):

> If they just can't wait ... before I end up with a child who gets a STD, or gets someone pregnant, I would have to get them birth control. I worry more about my son, if he gets someone pregnant you would have to deal with her and her family. If I have to put a bowl of condoms out there—maybe he'd be mortified enough by having his father teach him how to use it—but I don't want him to have a child and become a deadbeat dad.

Among those with strong religious beliefs, parents were likely to say that they were teaching their sons and daughters abstinence, but overall there was still the tendency to police the sexuality of daughters more than that of sons. Sons are more likely to be taught to use protection rather than to avoid sex. As one mother of a 16-year-old son said:

> I buy him condoms—and I am very, very worried about his sexuality, as far as being safe, more than his sexuality. I buy condoms and he lets me know that he's out or getting low—I don't know if he gives them to his friends, which is fine with me. He says he's not doing it [having sex], but I'm a mother, and I know better.

Teenage sexuality has declined in recent years and the use of contraceptives has increased, leading to a decline in teenage pregnancy. Still, such pregnancies are more common among those who are low-income and African American. Teenage sexuality is not inherently harmful or "risky," although some might argue that most teenagers are not mature enough to fully understand the social and emotional implications of sexual intimacy. This is even more likely when they engage in casual sex during transient relationships or are coerced into sexual relationships.

Beyond sex education

Sex education and birth control are important for reducing the adverse consequences of sex among teenagers. But initiation into sexual activity is not always voluntary or consensual, especially for girls, and social inequality heightens those risks. Much of the risky sexual behavior that goes on is the result of coercive sexual relationships that occur because girls lack adequate supervision, have little power over their own lives, are drug or substance-dependent, or are mired in lives of poverty that make them indifferent to the risks of STDs and even pregnancy. Rape and coercive sexuality are too common, and low-income black girls are the most common victims. As one of my respondents explained:

> You know, I had a STD before. I was 16 and still in high school, 16-17, something like that, I don't remember. I had a time where I was raped. I didn't tell for two weeks but then it came out ... so after that situation I had to go to the

> doctors and get all these tests. One was about pregnancy ...
> my son wasn't my first pregnancy. He was my first live birth.

More common than rape is being coerced into having sex. Female teenagers are often at a disadvantage in sexual encounters, especially since males usually have more power, are often older, and are socialized to be more sexually aggressive. Black girls are more likely than white girls to be inadequately supervised by their parents or living outside their parents' home, and are also more likely to be involved with older men, sexually abused, or otherwise involved in involuntary sex (Abma et al, 1998). Studies show that young females lack the decision-making power to negotiate sex with their partners or insist that they use condoms, even in consensual relations (Pflieger et al, 2013).

Teenage sexuality, whether based on coercion or consensus, carries considerable risks, but even more so for low-income African Americans. Fully half of African-American girls between the ages of 14 and 19 (compared to 20 percent of white female teenagers) have or have had a STD, and such diseases are linked to infertility and other health problems (Weitz, 2013). African-American teens account for 65 percent of HIV diagnoses among those aged between 13 and 24 (Jackson et al, 2015). Teenage sexuality is also associated with other health and social problems. One study of several hundred sexually active African-American teenage girls living in Georgia found that 40 percent had significant symptoms of depression and 65 percent had used an illegal substance during the past three months (Jackson et al, 2015).

The failure of teenagers to protect themselves from the risks of pregnancy has been the topic of numerous studies, with theories explaining the higher rate of early sexuality among African Americans as the result of a lack of sex education and reduced access to birth control. Many have found that low-income females are likely to become pregnant more because of indifference than desire to be mothers, although the latter may play a part. Most do not see having children during their teenage years or outside of marriage as preferable, but neither do they see it as stigmatizing or precluding other life options. Life opportunities (or the lack thereof) shape attitudes about sex and childbearing. Browning et al, for example, found neighborhood disadvantage to be an important factor in more liberal attitudes towards sex and childbearing among young people (Browning et al, 2008).

Life opportunities and the chances that teenagers perceive themselves as having affect their likelihood of protecting themselves against pregnancy and STDs. Having high educational goals is often associated by rational choice theorists as a motivating factor in avoiding risky sexual behaviors and pregnancy. But analyzing data from the National Educational Longitudinal Study, one study found that inflated educational expectations and low actual achievement creates a mismatch between educational expectations and achievement that actually increases the risk of unprotected sex among adolescents. One reason is that the mismatch leads to shame and guilt–social psychological processes that undermine self-regulation (Beattie, 2015).

Childrearing: a race–class perspective

Most parents love their children and do their best to take care of them. Most invest heavily in their children, whether measured in time, money, or emotions. And the parents of young children across social class boundaries are optimistic about their children's futures. But economic resources matter a lot in childhood outcomes, and parents who are economically disadvantaged simply do not have as much to invest in their children. Children in the US run a high risk of growing up in poor and low-income households. One in every five children in the nation, and slightly more than 60 percent of black children, live in economically disadvantaged families. Poverty rates for children are higher than those for adults: children make up 25 percent of the population, but 41 percent of those living in low-income families. Countless numbers of children who grow up poor go on to succeed in life, for example, they get jobs, marry, start families, and many even experience socioeconomic mobility. But overall they do not experience the same success as those who grow up in more economically affluent households.

One reason is that social class shapes parenting strategies. Evidence for the importance of social class dates back to research conducted in the 1950s, which found distinct differences in the ways that working- and middle-class parents socialize their children. Parents instilled in their children the values important for success in their own occupational worlds; for example, those in the working class emphasized obedience and respect for authority, while those in the middle class emphasized things like autonomy and creativity (Kohn, 1963). Annette Lareau and her colleagues have more recently elaborated on this research. Social class, they argued, shapes the cultural logic parents used in rearing their children. Middle- and upper-class parents engage in concerted cultivation, characterized by a busy, highly organized schedule of daily activities, the extensive use of language, and an emphasis on social connections. Less affluent parents—those in the working and lower classes—engage in accomplishment by natural growth. Children have more time for informal activities, such as watching television and hanging out with relatives. These parents did not verbally interact with their children as much, and were less likely to explain things or negotiate with their children (Lareau, 2003). Each strategy has benefits and costs, but the long-term effects were that middle- and upper-class children grew up with a sense of entitlement, were better able to navigate the educational system and labor market, and more likely to experience career success. Thus, parental practices play an important role in the perpetuation of social inequality across generations.

Social class has a more powerful influence than race on parents' childrearing strategies, but African-American parents face the additional responsibility of racially socializing their children. Regardless of social class, black children grow up in a society where blackness signifies inferiority, and all too often their living conditions reinforce that message. By racially socializing their children, parents hope to prepare them for the possibility of being treated unfairly because of their race and teach them how to respond to racism. Black children also often compare themselves unfavorably to white children in terms of physical appearance and lifestyle, and racial socialization aims to address those issues by instilling racial and cultural pride in children.

Motherhood and poverty

Beyond childrearing strategies, being born to low-income parents and growing up in poverty exposes children to numerous health risks, often from the moment of conception. In 2009 the Centers for Disease Control and Prevention reported that about 29 percent of African-American women (and 11 percent of white women) do not get prenatal care during the first trimester of their pregnancies, a racial gap resulting from the facts that black mothers, on average, are younger, poorer, and less likely to be insured. Black children face more health challenges than white children from the moment of birth, often due to having higher rates of preterm delivery and low birth weight (Rosenthal and Lobel, 2011). Analyzing data from the California Maternal and Infant Health Assessment Survey, Braveman and colleagues found that preterm birth deliveries among women living in households with incomes at or below the poverty level were three times higher for black than for white mothers. All of these women experienced economic hardship, but the level of poverty was deeper for black women and amplified by stress and racial discrimination. Low birth weight predicts a host of developmental challenges, which are compounded by risk factors in the environment, such as exposure to lead poisoning that comes from the lead-based paint used in older homes and neighborhoods (Braveman et al, 2015).

Poor mothers often have their own health issues, and there is a connection between the health of mothers and their children. For example, mothers who experience depression are much more likely to have children with depression, and mothers who have children with disabilities and functional limitations have more adverse physical and mental outcomes (Garbarski, 2014). Studies have shown that parental stress, which is higher in single-mother families, also diminishes the ability of parents to tend to the emotional and psychological needs of their children. One result is that poor children have more externalizing and aggressive behaviors (Mackler et al, 2015), and inherit a health disadvantage that lasts throughout life (Umberson et al, 2014).

Low-income households experience more family instability, even more so if they are headed by single mothers (McLanahan and Schwartz, 2002; McLanahan and Percheski, 2008; Alexander et al, 2014). Geographic mobility accounts for some of the problems faced by children, as poor families are often forced to relocate due to evictions and other housing problems, leaving children to adapt to new neighborhoods, teachers, schools, and peer networks. Federal subsidies for housing have fallen significantly in recent decades, as has the supply of housing for the poor, and even those who qualify for housing subsidies are often on long wait lists.

Constantly relocating often means that the composition of the household children grow up in changes frequently, as families evade homelessness by moving in with friends and relatives. In many cases, the living conditions are overcrowded, affording little privacy, and routines such as regular mealtimes and bedtimes are absent. In his interviews with low-income black men, Alford Young reported that, asked to describe the households they grew up in, many were unable to do so. Describing the families they grew up in, Young explained:

> Crises and uncertainties were common features of family life. Relatives came and went regularly over the years as a response to the loss of a job, the inability to pay rent, or the need to avoid a threatening or problematic resident in their own domicile.... The birth and departure of siblings throughout their childhood, coupled with the temporary (but sometimes extremely lengthy) household hosting of

aunts, uncles, and cousins, made family life an unstable, if not altogether turbulent, experience. (Young, 2004: 72-3)

An ever-shifting household composition can also result from cohabitation and multipartner fertility. Unmarried parents are often involved in a series of cohabitating relationships, leaving their children to adjust to several male or female partners along with halfsiblings and stepsiblings who are in their lives only temporarily. About 60 percent of children born to unmarried parents have a halfsibling or stepsibling, and emerging research shows that by the time they enter school these children have higher levels of anxiety and aggressiveness (Fomby et al, 2015). Children living with cohabitating parents have about a 75 percent chance of seeing one of their parents leave the household before they reach the age of 15 (Cherlin, 2009), and those parents often go on to have children with other partners, further complicating family relations. One study reported that 8 percent of American men between the ages of 15-44 have children by more than one women, but more than one-third of poor black men aged 35-44 do, and 16 percent have children with three or more women (Guzzo and Furstenberg, 2007). These transitions also diminish the family's material resources, increase maternal stress, and reduce the quality of mothering (Osborne and McLanahan, 2007).

For decades researchers have pointed out that ineffective parenting and child abuse and neglect are disproportionately found among the poor. African-American parents are more likely to engage in authoritarian or power-assertive childrearing strategies, for example, expecting instant obedience to strict rules, demanding respect, and using physical punishment (Nomaguchi and House, 2013). Many middle-class African-American parents support spanking their children based on their own upbringing and religious beliefs. But poverty and hardship create psychological distress and diminish the ability of parents to be patient with and sensitive to their children. African-American children are overpresented among victims of child abuse and neglect in the child welfare system. They are more likely to be removed from their homes for abuse and less likely to return, and their high rates of behavioral and psychological problems often means they wait longer for placement in foster homes (Anyon, 2011).

Family structure and children's health

The past decade has seen considerable debate over the impact of family structure—usually single-mother families—on poverty, health, and children. The weight of evidence suggests that children growing up in married-couple families composed of both their biological parents have a health advantage over children in other families. The most obvious reason is that two-parent families usually have two wage earners and more resources for creating a stable family life. Raising a child requires the efforts of at least two people, whether they are the biological parents or not, and this is even more the case today with parents who are trying to balance family and employment. Asked to name what caused them the most stress, it is not surprising that the single most common stressor for single parents was paying the bills (41 percent) and the second most common was poor health (38 percent) (Eamon and Wu, 2011). Most mothers are employed, and day care has never been as available or affordable as it could be. This scarcity of reliable childcare is made worse by the current 24/7 economy since many parents, but especially low-income parents, work hours when most day care centers are closed.

One of my respondents, Lacy, is a 31-year-old single mother of a five-year-old son, and they are currently living with her grandmother. She describes herself as a loner and fairly isolated. Lacy would really like to accept a job as a home health care worker—she has an offer of work, but does not have anyone to take care of her son:

> I feel isolated, more so like being a single parent and not having the proper help. It gets difficult, I mean, for me it is difficult because if I get a job offer at a certain time I can't take it because I don't have that support with my son. I have a job offer from 3 to 11 shift, but I wouldn't know what to do with my son. I want to take it, but I'm still trying to find someone to keep my son.... I am living with my grandmother, but she's 80 years old, and it might be too much for her.

Many employed parents have no reliable, consistent source of childcare, and children are passed from home to home, where eating, sleeping, and household rules vary. This may explain why single mothers in general are twice as likely as married mothers to be unemployed, and are more likely to have short-term, low-paying jobs with inadequate benefits.

There are obvious reasons why family structure may be related to childhood outcomes, but the topic warrants a few caveats. One is the growing complexity, diversity, and fluidity of families regardless of whether they are headed by one or two parents. Single-parent families almost always invoke images of low-income welfare-dependent mothers and their children, but single-parent families are increasingly racially and economically diverse, and some are headed by single fathers. Not all single-parent families are on the economic margins, nor are all married-couple families affluent or immune from the stress, conflict, and deprivation associated with poor health outcomes. Families are also very fluid, due to high rates of divorce, remarriage, and nonmarital cohabitation. Children may live a portion of their lives with grandparents or other relatives, or with same-sex parents. These family structures may change over the course of children's lives, making it difficult to describe what kind of family they "grew up" in. Moreover, family structure is a proxy for other social and economic factors that affect health, such as stress, social isolation, parenting quality, access to health care, and the entire broader context of life that shapes health.

Father absence

Increasing rates of divorce and nonmarital childbearing have made fathers' presence in the lives of their children a major political issue. Nearly half of new marriages end in divorce, and 40 percent of children are born to single parents. Much of the concern about missing fathers was motivated by the growth of welfare dependency among single mothers. Welfare reform included a Responsible Fatherhood Act that aimed to teach low-income men how to form successful marriages and encourage them to provide economically for their children; however, it neglected to offer much along the lines of employment opportunities or job training. Scholars agree that fathers are important and have devoted more research to exploring how they contribute to the lives of their children beyond their provider roles.

Father-absent families have been a longstanding issue in discussions about the welfare of African Americans, where single-mother families have always been prevalent. Nearly 70 percent of black children are born to single parents, and many will spend most or all of their childhood in a single-mother family. Households with nonresidential fathers now transcend racial and social class boundaries, but most research shows that the consequences of growing up without a father in the home are the same for all children, for example, poorer academic performance, more externalizing behavior among boys, and more early sex and pregnancy among girls (McLanahan and Schwartz, 2002). Still, the comparison of father-absent with father-present homes is challenging in several ways, most basically in the assumption that fathers who live with their children are actively involved in their lives but nonresidential fathers are not. Fathers can be marginal figures in their children's lives, even when they are married to their children's mother. Asked to describe the family she grew up in, one of my interviewees said:

> I wouldn't say I grew up in a single-parent home—I had my dad, he was kind of in and out. My mom and dad were married, but he was out of the house a lot because of the job he chose and the kind of lifestyle he had. It was probably some illegal stuff, and then he always ended up in prison … but [my dad] was in and out until he passed, about 10 years ago. He has a massive heart attack, complications from diabetes, they said. He was 53 years old.

Most nonresidential fathers are at least somewhat involved with their children. One 47-year-old never-married father of four children I interviewed lives in close proximity to his children, spends a great deal of time with them, and considers himself a good father:

> I was 18 when I became a father. Birth of my first child, [it] was great. I enjoyed it. I was happy. I felt ready to be a father, but my life wasn't in order yet. You have to make the best of it, to do what you gotta do. I have three additional children, all with the same mother. I'm tough, I'm hard, I'm strict—I think I'm a good father. I don't want them to fall and make the same mistakes I did. I have their best interests at heart; they don't know what this world is like.

The extent to which children are adversely impacted by having a nonresidential father varies based on whether their father ever lived in the household, how often he visits, how much time they spend with him, and the availability of other father figures.

None of this denies the adverse behavioral outcomes related to growing up without a father in home, but rather suggests that many factors mediate those outcomes. Nor does it ignore the fact that children whose fathers are uninvolved or minimally involved in their lives experience a lot of emotional and psychological distress. Black magazines such as *Ebony and Essence* have published many essays from

adult children, mostly men, who grew up having little or no contact with their fathers. Most have high praise for their mothers and the other women who reared them, but uniformly describe a childhood filled with disappointment as they struggled to understand why their fathers seemed so disinterested in them. Some have other men in their lives who offer advice, encourage, and support—"other daddies" (Haney and March, 2003)—but rarely are they able to develop a stable, consistent, and lasting relationship with them. The absence of a relationship with one's own biological father can cause a great deal of distress for children. Joyce Macy is in her 60s and has had a successful career. Asked about her growing up experiences, she described her father this way:

> Yes, I knew [my father], but I didn't like him. I didn't like him because he would promise us things but wouldn't follow through. He would tell our mother he was going to come pick us up, me and my brother ... we'd be sitting in the front couch, wanting to go out and play but we couldn't because she had cleaned us up. But he wouldn't show.

Once Joyce's son was born, her father started trying to connect with her: "he wanted me to call him 'daddy' and I told him I'm not going to do that." She went on to say:

> Then he was really sick and he called me and he asked me for help, because he knew he was going to the hospital ... and probably wouldn't be coming out.... I said 'no.' Then he went there and died and I feel really bad about that. I was 28 years old. He had blood clots of something. It's really bad because I just dismissed him—that's terrible, huh?

Intergenerational kin support

When I arrived at Mildred's house, she apologized for having three grandchildren on hand; their mother had suddenly become ill and had to be taken to the emergency room. Mildred is not yet 60 but has been retired for several years due to multiple health issues, so she is often the go-to babysitter for the three of her four children who have children. On most days Mildred has at least two or three grandchildren on hand, but it is difficult to say how many she has, especially if one goes by biological ties. Her oldest daughter has two children with two different fathers, both of whom also have fathered children with other women.

Should they be counted as her grandchildren? An unmarried son has three children; a second son, Cameron, has at least two children by different women—perhaps a third. As Mildred explained, "the DNA is still out on that one." Cameron has only recently been released from prison and still has drug addiction issues. His relationship with his current girlfriend is extremely tense: she had three children before meeting Cameron, and they have one together. She had a fourth one while he was in prison, but gave it up for adoption because the child was fathered by another man. Thus, Mildred has several children who may or may not be counted as her grandchildren.

I describe these details to highlight the complexities of many families and one of the reasons intergenerational kin support has waned. Mildred generously helps out with her grandchildren and quasi-grandchildren as much as she can, but they strain her limited resources. Providing assistance is also complicated by the tensions her children experience with the various partners they have had over the years, and the fact that Mildred's own health is marginal. She has survived intimate partner violence and drug addiction, but struggles with a host of chronic health issues that frequently land her in the hospital.

Intergenerational kin networks are cited as one of the strengths of African-American families; indeed, it is difficult to understand black families without considering extended family ties. Fathers were often absent, many agreed, but black mothers could not really be defined as "single" because they had the support of a strong kinship network (mostly other women) who stepped in to help with childrearing. Extended family networks may be rooted in African traditions, but were reinforced during slavery when mothers could often not care for their own children. In his early work, Frazier described black grandmothers as "guardians of the generations," as they helped raise children whose mothers had to work and stood in for absent fathers (Frazier, 1957). In many cases black grandmothers functioned more like mothers, playing a central role in providing discipline and training for children, and other female relatives pitched in to help. This has led some black feminists to argue that motherhood is organized differently among African-American women, as a collective rather than a private responsibility, with "other mothers" playing a vital role in assisting biological mothers with their children (Collins, 1990). Extended family ties are still strong in most African-American families, but often the single mothers who need help the most are not beneficiaries of much support.

The economic and family crises of the 1970s, along with greater class diversity and mobility among black families, significantly strained the resiliency of extended family networks. The rate of pregnancy for young single black teenage females escalated and, given the trend of intergenerational teenage pregnancy, grandmothers were sometimes barely in their 30s. By the 1980s, Ladner and Gourdine—scholars who once described single-mother black families as functional and shaped by the African cultural traditions—wrote:

> [Black] grandmothers complain about their own unmet emotional and social needs. They appear to feel powerless in coping with the demands made by their children. They comment frequently that their children show them no respect, do not listen to their advice, and place little value on their roles as parents. (Ladner and Gourdine, 1984: 23)

Those who start childbearing at an earlier age have an overall higher fertility rate than those who do not, and both they and their partners are more likely to have children with other partners. This now common pattern of childbearing complicates kinship bonds and obligations and diminishes support from grandparents. Many are willing to help with their own biological grandchildren, but not with other children living in the same household with them.

Although they have emotional ties to their grandchildren and want to be involved in their lives, most grandparents do not want the responsibility of providing the basic essentials children need or becoming primary caregivers. Nevertheless, many grandparents whose resources are already strained find themselves called up to help support their grandchildren. In many cases, this means living in multigenerational households: between 2011-13, the percentage of the population over 30 and living in an extended family setting was 5.9 percent for Blacks compared to 2.6 percent for Whites (Coles, 2016). In other cases, grandparents are completely responsible for the care of their grandchildren because their adult sons and daughters are incarcerated, homeless, drug- or alcohol-dependent, or simply unable to provide for their children. By 2014, these "skipped generation" households were slightly more common among African Americans (28 percent) than Whites (24 percent) (Coles, 2016).

Some grandparents may take pride in being able to help raise their grandchildren, but many who take on the responsibility lack the resources needed to raise children. Even those who are young are often dealing with their own health issues. One 52-year-old grandmother I interviewed who lives in public housing and retired early because of her own health issues now finds herself rearing two of her grandsons, both of whom have chronic illnesses. She described her daughter, the mother of the children, as "foot-loose and fancy free," but tried to put a positive spin on the responsibility of caring for her grandchildren:

> My being ill—and now instead of playing the role of grandmother, playing the role of mother—I think it helps me personally with my own illness because of the fact that it keeps me on my toes. Even when I don't feel like it, I have to push myself to take care of them.... I can't let my boys down; I have to continue to push myself to do things for them. I can't let them look at me and say, 'Momma's sick.' I don't know why in the world the Lord would let this happen ... maybe the Lord did this and let it all fall off on me to keep me having something to strive for and keep my own self alive. (quoted in Hill, 1994)

The availability of social support and its impact on families is an important issue, especially given substantial evidence that it mediates the stress of economic and emotional difficulties. People of all racial groups have family members they can call on for various types of assistance, but there are racial and class dimensions of that support. Ann Rochelle was one of the first to compare black and white families and to find that black families were no more likely than white families—and often less likely—to provide various forms of social support to their members (Roschelle, 1997). More recent research also finds that black and white families have different patterns of kin involvement, with African Americans providing more practical support such as child care and help with transportation, and Whites more financial and emotional support (Sarkisian and Gerson, 2004).

Social class inequalities more than cultural traditions account for extended family support. Poor mothers are often less likely to be able to access social support, since their networks tend to be composed of other poor people who are not in a good position to offer emotional or economic support. Some of these mothers end up relying on their own children for support, which has been shown to have an adverse impact on the children's health (Mickelson and Demmings, 2009). Social support from kin is stronger when it is voluntary and reciprocal, but more problematic when people are called on to help relatives who always seem on the brink of a crisis.

Social support can also be a double-edged sword, both easing and elevating stress. Although social isolation can increase depression, for example, people who are isolated from stressful family relationships have lower levels of stress, anger, and agitation (Ross and Mirowsky,

2009). Financial strains are especially associated with more negative interactions with relatives and higher rates of depression, especially for single black women (Lincoln et al, 2005). Life course theory suggests a stage in life when the children are launched into the world and parents are free to devote their time to careers and other activities. But in many cases, black grandparents are unable to extricate themselves from the demands of providing care for adult children and grandchildren. These responsibilities make the middle years stressful and more difficult for them to take care of their own health needs. This may help explain why black people carry a health deficit into their middle and later years.

Neighborhoods, schools, and health

In November 2015 nine-year-old Tyshawn Lee was on his way to visit his grandmother on the South Side of Chicago when he stopped at a playground along the way. He was lured off the playground by a man who offered to buy him something at a store, but instead took him into an alley and shot him several times at close range. The 22-year-old African-American male who did this was assisted by two fellow gang members, who arrived shortly thereafter to help clean up the mess. The murder was motivated by revenge: Tyshawn's father was the member of a gang that had been accused of killing the brother of one of three men who planned the boy's death. The original plan called for kidnapping Tyshawn and torturing him by cutting off his fingers and ears, but in the end, they decided to just shoot him. One of Tyshawn's assailants, whose mother had been wounded and brother had been shot to death in gang warfare, had vowed to avenge these assaults by killing "grandmas, mamas, kids, and all" in the future (Casbillo and Martinez, 2016).

The entire community, including police officers, were horrified at the sinister nature of the crime—brutally killing a nine-year-old as revenge for the actions of his father. Children are not usually targeted for murder, although it is not uncommon for them to be caught in the crosshairs of the gang warfare and crime wave that is sweeping across many cities. In 2011 6,309 African Americans were victims of homicide and 8 percent of them—487 children, some of them quite young—were among those victims (Sugarmann, 2014). African-American boys living in cities at the age of 16 have only a 50 to 62 percent chance of surviving to the age of 65, compared to an 80 percent chance for white boys living in similar situations (Martin et al, 2015). The prospect of early death due to homicide, and the distress and fear it invokes, is one of the most devastating effects of living in some poor urban neighborhoods.

Neighborhoods characterized by violence and poverty are strongly associated with adverse behavioral and health outcomes for African Americans in general, but especially male children. Black children from low-income households have high rates of aggressive acts and involvement in crime. In 2008, for example, black children accounted for 16 percent of the youth population, but were involved in 52 percent of all juvenile violent crime arrests in the US (Romero et al, 2015). But there are other health damaging consequences of living in disadvantaged neighborhoods, such as exposure to environmental risks, inadequate housing, lead poisoning, pollution, and toxins that impair brain development and the capacity for reasoning and decision-making.

These high-risk neighborhoods not only jeopardize children's lives and health, but they also shape their social, gender, and racial identities. Poor black children living in high-risk neighborhoods believe they have to fight for their own physical survival, or at least develop a tough persona. For children between the ages of 12-17, African Americans run a greater risk of witnessing violence at every income level than their white counterparts. Exposure to violence leads to aggressive behavior and psychological distress, affecting adolescent girls in particular (Mitchell et al, 2010). They learn that anyone can be the victim of a crime or street violence, even a child, and girls and boys are often encouraged by their parents to stand up for themselves. One survey of junior high school girls living in a poor, racially segregated area of New York City found that more than one-third had recently been involved in fights, weapon carrying, or weapon use, and more than one-half had threatened others with violence (Stueve et al, 2001). Unlike in the past, today's teenagers are less likely to be arrested for status offenses, such as skipping school, and more likely to be arrested for violent criminal offenses. Those arrested for violence share some common background experiences, for example, most live in poverty, in drug-abusing families, and have experienced sexual or physical abuse.

Schools in some poor neighborhoods offer little refuge from the violence and disorder that are found in neighborhoods; they are noisy, disorderly, and prone to violent eruptions. It is not surprising that children find it difficult to learn. One study of schools in large cities with populations of more than 250,000 found that by the fourth grade only 11 percent of black boys (compared to 38 percent of white boys) were reading at grade level (Chiles, 2013). African-American students bring into the classroom more behavioral and learning problems, and teachers often treat them according to the racial stereotype of black children as less intelligent and more likely to engage in disruptive behavior. In her ethnography of fifth and sixth grade students at a public elementary school, Ann Ferguson found that teachers were especially likely to racially stereotype black boys. While misbehaving white boys were described as engaging in normal childhood antics, black boys were likely to be labeled as "hypersexual, shiftless, lazy, and of inferior intellect," and destined for prison (Ferguson, 2000). Black children have considerably more detentions, suspensions, and special education placements than white children.

Environmental risk factors and racial stereotypes also shape the self-esteem and identity of black girls. In *Between good and ghetto*, Nikki Jones (2010) described the challenges black girls encounter in forging race and gender identities that enable them to survive in high-risk environments. The esteem of black children, but especially girls, is often diminished early in life when they realize that they do not meet Eurocentric standards of "beauty." From an early age, many show a preference for light skin and straight hair, and parents try to redefine standards of beauty and socialize their children into self-acceptance. Many try to teach their daughters to conform to conventional gender behaviors but also how to survive in rough neighborhoods, which is not easy. As Jones found in her ethnography, the number one concern is often self-protection. This means that black girls are often compelled to craft identities of toughness or strength, although doing so leaves them vulnerable to being described by others as "ghetto." Their race and gender identities are also affected by the hip-hop culture, where females are constantly imaged as "bitches and hos, gold diggers, hoodrats, ghetto chicks [and] ride-or-die bitches" (Jones, 2010: 49). The psychological distress they experience during childhood makes them especially vulnerable to depression during their adult years (Rossin-Slater, 2015).

Conclusion

African-American parents across social classes lines invest heavily in their children, but vary a great deal in parenting strategies and resources. Black families are economically diverse, and not all children are poor or living in families and neighborhoods that are high-risk. Many live in married-couple, two-parent, middle-class households with parents who are as likely as their white counterparts to invest heavily in their children. But the majority of black children live in low-income families and poverty, and this exposes them to multiple physical, emotional, and psychological disadvantages. Children who live in poor and distressed families and neighborhoods are two to four times more likely to have a disease than children who do not (Rossin-Slater, 2015). One recent alarming statistic has been the increased rate of suicide for young black children between the ages of five and eleven. Between 1993 and 2012, the rate of suicide for black children in this age range increased by more than 150 percent, while those for white children fell by half (Tavernise, 2015). Experiencing childhood adversities has implications that stretch into adulthood. Growing up in poverty and on welfare has been found to predict higher levels of psychological distress and lower self-esteem for women (Engsminger, 1995), and manifests itself over the life course in increased substance abuse, more heart attacks, depression, and functional limitations (Pavalko and Caputo, 2013). On the other hand, the prospects of intergenerational mobility for children are greatly improved when their parents move into better neighborhoods. One recent study found that when low-income parents are able to move to better neighborhoods, their children achieve more in school and have higher earnings as adults (Johnson, 2016).

The US provides an array of health and social programs designed to support low-income families and children, such as nutrition and early education programs, housing subsidies, and health insurance. Health care expenditures for children have grown in recent decades, mostly because the declining economic standing of families has made more people eligible for public health care programs. This increase in public expenditures on children's health, however, has come with a loss in public investment for other social services, such as education and housing assistance (Rossin-Slater, 2015).

Although access to health care is important for families and children, it matters less than other social factors, such as their family life, poverty, and the social environment in which they live (Leininger and Levy, 2015). Improving the health of black children requires addressing the issues of poverty and inequitable distribution of resources in schools and neighborhoods.

Conclusion

This book has focused on how race and racism affect sickness and mortality among African Americans. Social conditions and economic inequality are now widely accepted as the major causes of sickness and premature death. Numerous social conditions adversely affect health, including poor living conditions, stressful work environments, and strained family and social relationships. Most of these social conditions are the result of economic inequalities, which have grown dramatically in the US during the past few years. High levels of income inequality within nations predict worse health in the population (Pickett and Wilkinson, 2015), and the US has a higher level of income inequality than other Western nations. Moreover, millions of Americans still lack health insurance, despite recent health care reform policies. These inequalities help account for the fact that the US ranks lower than other advanced nations on basic indicators of population health, such as infant mortality and average life span. A college-educated, white, upper-middle class American who practices good health behaviors is, on average, in worse health than his counterparts in comparable industrialized nations (Gilligan, 2015).

Within the US, racial disparities in health have remained stark: Blacks have higher rates of sickness and infant mortality than other races, and the shortest life spans. Black rates of poverty and joblessness are more than twice that for Whites, and black people often live in poor neighborhoods and occupy low-level jobs in the labor market. These social and economic inequalities, however, often mask the significance of race and racism in shaping health outcomes. Racial stereotypes, exclusion, and discrimination are chronic stressors and take a toll on black health. Institutionalized racism operates in less visible ways to undermine health, such as less spending on public services in black neighborhoods, targeting African Americans for risky housing loans, and racial discrepancies in criminal sentencing. The adverse effects of these policies are compounded in a society that emphasizes social mobility through hard work yet offers limited opportunities for the disadvantaged to achieve that mobility. Failure is often internalized, resulting in what Emirbayer and Desmond (2015) have called symbolic violence, the "misrecognizing oneself as something less than a full individual—as something less than a person entitled to dignities, protections, and rights—and thus resigning oneself to a kind of partial and unfulfilled humanity" (Emirbayer and Desmond, 2015: 264).

The contradiction between the ideology of equal opportunity for all races and the persistence of seemingly intractable inequalities has consequences for the entire nation. Sickness and early death drive up the cost of medical care and lower overall economic productivity. The nation's poor health outcomes reflect racial and class inequalities in access to health care and decent living conditions, and tarnishes the reputation of its medical system and its image as a world leader. It fosters racially divisive theories to explain why some groups are more successful than others, and leaves the nation spending billions of dollars to manage restive populations, social protest, and crime. These problems—and the pursuit of simple justice—have made eliminating racial disparities in health a persistent slogan among public health advocates and the goal of federal initiatives such as Healthy People. This goal cannot be achieved by rhetoric challenging racist ideologies, but rather the more demanding task of altering the underlying social structural inequalities that foster racial inequalities.

References

Abma, Joyce, Anne Driscoll and Kristin Moore. 1998. "Young women's degree of control over first intercourse: An exploratory analysis." *Family Planning Perspectives* 30(1): 12-18.

Abraham, Laurie Kaye. 1993. *Mama might be better off dead: The failure of health care in urban America.* Chicago, IL: University of Chicago Press.

Aday, Ron H. and Jennifer J. Krabill. 2011. *Women aging in prison: A neglected population in the correctional system.* Boulder, CO: Lynne Rienner Publishers.

Aholou, Tiffiany M., Eric Cooks, Ashley Murray, Madeline Y. Sutton, Zaneta Gaul, Susan Gaskins and Pamela Payne-Foster. 2016: forthcoming. "'Wake up! HIV is at your door': African American faith leaders in the rural south and HIV perceptions: A qualitative analysis." *Journal of Religion and Health.*

Alexander, Karl, Doris Entwisle and Linda Olson. 2014. *The long shadow: Family background, disadvantaged urban youth, and the transition to adulthood.* New York: Russell Sage Foundation.

Alexander, Michelle. 2010. *The new Jim Crow: Mass incarceration in the age of colorblindness.* New York: The New Press.

Anyon, Yolanda. 2011. "Reducing racial disparities and disproportionalities in the child welfare system: Policy perspectives about how to serve the best interests of African American youth." *Children and Youth Services Review* 33(2): 242-53.

Armstrong, Katrina, Karima Ravenell, Suzanne McMurphy and Mary Putt. 2007. "Racial/ethnic differences in physician distrust in the United States." *American Journal of Public Health* 97(7): 1283-89.

Aronson, Joshua, Diana Burgess, Sean M. Phelan and Lindsay Juarez. 2013. "Unhealthy interactions: The role of stereotype threat in health disparities." *American Journal of Public Health* 103(1): 50-6.

Atherly, Adam and Karoline Mortensen. 2014. "Medicaid primary care physician fees and the use of preventive services among Medicaid enrollees." *Health Services Research* 49(4): 1306-28.

Bahr, Peter Riley. 2007. "Race and nutrition: An investigation of Black-White differences in health-related nutritional behaviours." *Sociology of Health & Illness* 29(6): 831-56.

Baker, R. B., H. A. Washington, O. Olakanmi, T. L. Savitt, E. A. Jacobs, E. Hoover and M. K. Wynia. 2008. "African American physicians and organized medicine, 1846-1968: Origins of a racial divide." *Journal of the American Medical Association* 300(3): 306-13.

Bankole, Katherine. 1998. *Slavery and medicine: Enslavement and medical practices in Antebellum Louisiana.* New York and London: Garland Publishing.

Banks, Ralph Richard. 2011. *Is marriage for White people? How African American marriage decline affects everyone.* New York: Dutton.

Baptist, Edward E. 2014. *The half has never been told: Slavery and the making of American capitalism.* New York: Basic Books.

Baptiste-Roberts, Kesha, Tiffany L. Gary, Gloria L. A. Beckles, Edward W. Gregg et al. 2007. "Family history of diabetes, awareness of risk factors, and health behaviors among African Americans." *American Journal of Public Health* 97(5): 907-12.

Barnes, Lisa L. 2014. "Alzheimer's disease in African Americans." *Health Affairs* 33(4): 580-86.

Barnes, Sandra L. 2013. *Live long and prosper : How Black megachurches address HIV/AIDS and poverty in the age of prosperity theology.* New York: Fordham University Press.

Barr, Ashley B., Elizabeth Culatta and Ronald L. Simons. 2013. "Romantic relationships and health among African American young adults: Linking patterns of relationship quality over time to changes in physical and mental health." *Journal of Health and Social Behavior* 54(3): 369–385.

Baum, Fran and Matthew Fisher. 2014. "Why behavioural health promotion endures despite its failure to reduce health inequities." *Sociology of Health & Illness* 36(2): 213-25.

Beardsley, Edward H. 1990. "Race as a factor in health." In R. D. Apple (ed) *Women, health, and medicine in America* (pp 121-42). New York: Garland Publishing, Inc.

Beattie, Irenee R. 2015. "Mismatched educational expectations and achievement and adolescent women's risk of unprotected first sex." *Sociological Perspectives* 58(3): 358-79.

Bennefield, Zinobia C. 2015. "Disparities in HPV and cervical cancer screening between highly educated white and minority young women." *American Journal of Health Education* 46: 90-8.

Bird, Chloe E. and Patricia P. Rieker. 2008. *Gender and health: The effects of constrained choices and social policies.* Cambridge, UK: Cambridge University Press.

Blodorn, Alison, Brenda Major and Cheryl Kaiser. 2016. "Perceived discrimination and poor health: Accounting for self-blame complicates a well-established relationship." *Social Science & Medicine* 153: 27-34.

Blount, Melissa. 1984. "Surpassing obstacles: Black women in medicine." *Journal of the American Medical Women's Association* 39(1): 192-5.

Boardman, Jason D., Jarron M. Saint Onge, Richard G. Rogers and Justin T. Denney. 2005. "Race differentials in obesity: The impact of place." *Journal of Health and Social Behavior* 46(3): 229-43.

Bobo, Lawrence, James R. Kluegel and Ryan A. Smith. 1997. "Laissez-faire racism: The crystallization of a kinder, gentler, antiblack ideology." In S. A. Tuch and J. K. Martin (eds) *Racical attitudes in the 1990s: Continuity and change* (pp 15-42). Westport, CT: Praeger.

Bonilla-Silva, Eduardo. 2012. "The invisible weight of whiteness: The racial grammar of everyday life in contemporary America." *Ethnic and Racial Studies* 35(2): 173-94.

Bratter, Jenifer L. and Bridget K. Gorman. 2011. "Is discrimination an equal opportunity risk? Racial experiences, socioeconomic status, and health status among Black and White adults." *Journal of Health and Social Behavior* 52(3): 365-82.

Braveman, Paula A., Katherine Heck, Susan Egerter, Kristen S. Marchi, Tyan Parker Dominguez, Catherine Cubbin, Kathryn Fingar, Jay A. Pearson and Michael Curtis. 2015. "The role of socioeconomic factors in black-white disparities in preterm birth." *American Journal of Public Health* 105(4): 694-702.

Brenner, M. Harvey. 1987. "Economic change, alcohol consumption and disease mortality in nine industrialized countries." *Social Science & Medicine* 25: 119-32.

Brewster, Karin L. 1994. "Race differences in sexual activity among adolescent women: The role of neighborhood characteristics." *American Sociological Review* 59 (June): 408-24.

Bridges, Judith S. and Ann Marie Orza. 1996. "Black and White employed mothers' role experience." *Sex Roles* 35(5/6): 337-85.

Britton, Dana M. 2011. *Gender of crime.* Lanham, MD: Rowman & Littlefield.

Brooks, Jesse. 2014. "Defeating AIDS is a civil rights issue." *Oakland Post*, January 22.

Brown, Diane R., Verna M. Keith, James S. Jackson and Lawrence E. Gary. 2003. "(Dis)respected and (dis)regarded: Experiences of racism and psychological distress." In D. Robinson-Brown and V. M. Keith (eds) *In and out of our right minds: The mental health of African-American women*. New York: Columbia University Press.

Browning, Christopher R., Lori A. Burrington, Tama Leventhal and Jeanne Brooks-Gunn. 2008. "Neighborhood structural inequality, collective efficacy, and sexual risk behavior among urban youth." *Journal of Health and Social Behavior* 49(3): 269-85.

Burdette, Amy M., Janet Weeks, Terrence D. Hill and Isaac W. Eberstein. 2012. "Maternal religious attendance and low birth weight." *Social Science & Medicine* 74: 1961-67.

Burton, Linda M., Eduardo Bonilla-Silva, Victor Ray, Rose Buckelew and Elizabeth Hordge Freeman. 2010. "Critical race theories, colorism, and the decade's research on families of color." *Journal of Marriage and Family* 72 (June): 440-59.

Bush-Baskette, Stephanie R. 1998. "The war on drugs as a war against Black women." In S. L. Miller (ed) *Crime control and women: Feminist implications of criminal justice policy* (pp 113-29). Thousand Oaks, CA: Sage.

Byrd, W. Michael and Linda A. Clayton. 2000. *An American health dilemma, Vol 1: A medical history of African Americans and the problem of race: Beginnings to 1900*. New York: Routledge.

Carnegie, Mary Elizabeth. 1985. "The path we tread." In D. C. Hine (ed) *Black women in the nursing profession* (pp 149-56). New York: Garland Publishing, Inc.

Carr, Deborah and Kristen W. Springer. 2010. "Advances in families and health research in the 21st century." *Journal of Marriage and Family* 72(3): 743-61.

Casbillo, Mariano and Michael Martinez. 2016. "Suspect weighed torture of Slain Tyshawn Lee, 9, prosecutors say" (www.cnn.com/2016/03/08/us/chicago-tyshawn-lee-murder-charges/)

Chatters, L. M., A. W. Nguyen and R. J. Taylor. 2014. "Religion and spirituality among older African Americans, Asians, and Hispanics." In K. Whitfield and T. Baker (eds) *Handbook of minority aging* (pp 82-100). New York: Springer.

Cherlin, Andrew J. 2009. *Marriage-go-round: The state of marriage and the family in America today*. New York: Alfred A. Knopf.

Cherlin, Andrew J. 2013. *Public and private families: An introduction*. New York: McGraw-Hill.

Chiles, Nick. 2013. "The state of Black boys." *Ebony* LXVIII(7): 122-27.

Ciribassi, Rebekah M. and Crystal L. Patil. 2016. "'We don't wear it on our sleeve': Sickle-cell disease and the (in)visible body in parts." *Social Science & Medicine* 148: 131–38.

Clarke, Averil Y. 2011. *Inequalities in love: College-educated Black women and the barriers to romance and family.* Durham, NC: Duke University Press.

Cloud, David H., Ernest Drucker, Angela Browne and Jim Parsons. 2015. "Public health and solitary confinement in the United States." *American Journal of Public Health* 105(1): 18–26.

Coates, Ta-Nehisi. 2015. "The black family in an age of mass incarceration." *The Atlantic*, October 15.

Cockerham, William C. 2016. *Medical sociology.* Upper Saddle River, NJ: Pearson.

Cohen, Phillip N. 2015. *The family: Diversity, inequality, and social change.* New York and London: W. W. Norton & Company.

Cole, Luke W. and Sheila R. Foster. 2001. *From the ground up: Environmental racism and the rise of the environmental justice movement.* New York and London: New York University Press.

Coles, Roberta L. 2016. *Race and family: A structural approach.* Lanham, MD: Rowman & Littlefield.

Collins, C. F. 1996. "Commentary on the health and social status of African-American women." In C. F. Collins (ed) *African-American women's health and social issues* (pp 1–13). Westport, CN: Auburn House.

Collins, Patricia Hill. 1990. *Black feminist thought: Knowledge, consciousness, and the politics of empowerment.* Boston, MA: Unwin Hyman.

Collins, Patricia Hill. 2004. *Black sexual politics: African Americans, gender, and the new racism.* New York and London: Routledge.

Comfort, Megan. 2008. *Doing time together: Love and family in the shadow of the prison.* Chicago, IL and London: University of Chicago Press.

Comfort, Megan, Olga Grinstead, Kathleen McCartney, Philippe Bourgois and Kelly Knight. 2005. "'You can't do nothing in this damn place': Sex and intimacy among couples with an incarcerated male partner." *Journal of Sex Research* 42(1): 3–12.

Conrad, Peter and Kristin K. Barker. 2010. "The social construction of illness: Key insights and policy implications." *Journal of Health and Social Behavior* 51(1 suppl): S67–S79.

Conrad, Peter and Joseph W. Schneider. 1980. *The medicalization of society: On the transformation of human conditions into treatable disorders.* St Louis, MO: Mosby.

Coontz, Stephanie. 2005. *Marriage, a history: From obedience to intimacy, or How love conquered marriage.* New York: Viking Penguin.

Cornwell, Erin York and Linda J. Waite. 2012. "Social network resources and management of hypertension." *Journal of Health and Social Behavior* 53(2): 215-31.

Deal, Stephanie B., Amanda C. Bennett, Kristin M. Rankin and James W. Collins. 2014. "The relation of age to low birth weight rates among foreign-born Black mothers: A population based exploratory study." *Ethnicity and Disease* 24(4): 413-17.

Deitch, Michelle and Michael B. Mushlin. 2016. "What's going on in our prisons?" *New York Times,* January 4.

Desmond, Matthew. 2016. *Evicted: Poverty and profit in the American city.* New York: Crown Publishers.

Dill, Bonnie Thornton. 1988. "Our mothers' grief: Racial ethnic women and the maintenance of families." *Journal of Family History* 13(4): 415-31.

DiMatteo, M. Robin, Carolyn B. Murray and Summer L. Williams. 2009. "Gender disparities in physician-patient communication among African American patients in primary care." *Journal of Black Psychology* 35(2): 204-27.

Diuguid, L. W. 2016. "Prison burdens women, families." *Kansas City Star,* 7A, January 20.

Dominguez, T. P., E. F. Strong, N. Krieger, M. W. Gillman and J. W. Rich-Edwards. 2009. "Differences in the self-reported racism experiences of US-born and foreign-born Black pregnant women." *Social Science & Medicine* 69: 258-65.

Downey, Liam and Marieke van Willigen. 2005. "Environmental stressors: The mental health impacts of living near industrial activity." *Journal of Health and Social Behavior* 46(3): 289-305.

Downs, Jim. 2012. *Sick from freedom: African-American illness and suffering during the Civil War and reconstruction.* New York: Oxford University Press.

Drake, Bruce. 2016. "Five facts about race in America." Washington, DC: Pew Research Center (www.pewresearch.org/fact-tank/2016/01/18/5-facts-about-race-in-america/).

Dutton, Diana B. 1978. "Explaining the low use of health services by the poor: Costs, attitudes, or delivery systems?" *American Sociological Review* 42(2): 348-68.

Eamon, Mary Keegan and Chi-Fang Wu. 2011. "Effects of unemployment and underemployment on material hardship in single-mother families." *Children and Youth Services Review* 33(2): 233-41.

Economist, The. 1989. "Crack babies." April 1.

Economist, The. 1990. "Goodbye, cocaine." September 8.

Edin, Kathryn. 2000. "What do low-income single mothers say about marriage?" *Social Problems* 47(1): 112-13.

Edin, Kathryn and Maria Kefalas. 2011. "Unmarried with children." In S. J. Ferguson (ed) *Shifting the center: Understanding contemporary families* (pp 725-32). New York: McGraw-Hill.

Ehrenreich, Barbara and Deirdre English. 1978. *For her own good: 150 years of expert advice to women.* Garden City, NY: Anchor Press.

Elder, Keith, Sudha Xirasagar, Nancy Miller, Shelly Ann Bowen, Saundra Glover and Crystal Piper. 2007. "African Americans' decisions not to evacuate New Orleans before Hurricane Katrina: A qualitative study." *American Journal of Public Health* 97(S1): S124-9.

Elliott, Sinika. 2012. *Not my kid: What parents believe about the sex lives of their teenagers.* New York: New York University.

Emirbayer, Mustafa and Matthew Desmond. 2015. *The racial order.* Chicago, IL and London: University of Chicago Press.

Engels, Friedrich. 1892 [1985]. *Origins of the family, private property, and the state.* Harmondsworth, UK: Penguin Books.

Engsminger, Margaret E. 1995. "Welfare and psychological distress: A longitudinal study of African American urban mothers." *Journal of Health and Social Behavior* 36 (December): 346-59.

Erving, Christy L. 2011. "Gender and physical health: A study of African American and Caribbean Black adults." *Journal of Health and Social Behavior* 52(3): 383-99.

Evans, Louwanda and Joe R. Feagin. 2015. "The costs of policing violence: Foregrounding cognitive and emotional labor." *Critical Sociology* 41(6): 887-95.

Faris, R. E. and H. W. Dunham. 1939. *Mental disorders in urban areas: An ecological study of schizophrenia and other psychoses.* Chicago, IL and London: University of Chicago Press.

Farley, John E. 2005. "Race, not class: Explaining racial housing segregation in the St Louis metropolitan area, 2000." *Sociological Focus* 38(2): 133-50.

Feagin, Joe and Zinobia Bennefield. 2014. "Systemic racism and US health care." *Social Science & Medicine* 103: 7-14.

Ferguson, Ann Arnett. 2000. *Bad boys: Public schools in the making of Black masculinity.* Ann Arbor, MI: University of Michigan Press.

Fletcher, Michael A. 2015. "White high school dropouts are wealthier than Black and Hispanic college grads." *Washington Post.* March 10.

Fomby, Paula, Joshua A. Goode and Stefanie Mollborn. 2015. "Family complexity, siblings, and children's aggressive behavior at school entry." *Demography* 53(1): 1-26.

Fontenot, Sarah Freyman. 2014. "Affordable Care Act: Lifting the curtain on health care costs." *Physician Executive Journal* (March–April): 78–81.

Franklin, Donna L. 1997. *Ensuring inequality: The structural transformation of the African-American family.* New York: Oxford University Press.

Franklin, Donna L. 2000. *What's love got to do with it? Understanding and healing the rift between Black men and women.* New York: Touchstone.

Frazier, E. Franklin. 1948. *The Negro family in the United States.* New York: Dryden Press.

Frazier, E. Franklin. 1957 [1939]. *The Negro in the United States.* New York: Macmillan.

Freidson, Eliot. 1960. "Client control and medical practice." *American Journal of Sociology* 65: 374–82.

Freidson, Eliot. 1970. *Profession of medicine: A study of the sociology of applied knowledge.* New York: Dodd, Mead.

Freimuth, Vicki S., Sandra Crouse Quinn, Stephen B. Thomas, Galen Cole, Eric Zook and Ted Duncan. 2001. "African Americans' views on research and the Tuskegee Syphilis Study." *Social Science & Medicine* 52: 797–808.

Frohlich, Katherine L. and Thomas Abel. 2014. "Environmental justice and health practices: Understanding how health inequities arise at the local level." *Sociology of Health and Illness* 36(2): 199–212

Garbarski, Dana. 2014. "The interplay between child and maternal health: Reciprocal relationships and cumulative disadvantage during childhood and adolescence." *Journal of Health and Social Behavior* 55(1): 91–106.

Garfield, R., R. Rudowitz, K. Young, L. Snyder, L. Clemans-Cope, E. Lawton and J. Holahan. 2015. *Trends in Medicaid spending leading up to ACA Implementation.* Kaiser Commission on Medicaid and the Uninsured.

Gengler, Amanda M. 2014. "'I want you to save my kid!': Illness management strategies, access, and inequality at an elite university research hospital." *Journal of Health and Social Behavior* 55(3): 342–59.

Gerhardt, Uta. 1989. *Ideas about illness: An intellectual and political history of medical sociology.* Washington Square, NY: New York University Press.

Geronimus, Arline. 2001. "Inequality in life expectany, functional status, and active life expectancy across selected black and white populations in the US." *Demography* 38(2): 227–51.

Gilbert, Dennis. 2011. *The American class structure in an age of growing inequality.* Thousand Oaks, CA: Sage Publications.

Gilligan, Heather Tirado. 2015. "Why racism is terrible for everyone's health." *JSTOR Daily*.

Glenn, Jason E. 2014. "Making crack babies: Race discourse and the biologization of behavior." In L. B. Green, J. McKiernan-Gonzalez and M. Summers (eds) *Precarious prescriptions: Contested histories of race and health in North America* (pp 237-60). Minneapolis, MN: University of Minnesota Press.

Gutman, Herbert G. 1976. *The Black family in slavery and freedom, 1750-1925*. New York: Pantheon.

Guzzo, Karen Benjamin and Frank F. Furstenberg. 2007. "Multipartnered fertility among American men." *Demography* 44(3): 583-601.

Guzzo, Karen Benjamin and Sarah R. Hayford. 2014. "Fertility and the stability of cohabiting unions: Variation by intendedness." *Journal of Family Issues* 35(4): 547-76.

Gwadz, Marya Viorst, Noelle Leonard, Charles Cleland, Marion Riedel, Angela Banfield and Donna Mildvan. 2011. "The effect of peer-driven intervention on rates of screening for AIDS clinical trials among African Americans and Hispanics." *American Journal of Public Health* 101(6): 1096-102.

Halfon, Neal. 2012. "Addressing health inequalities in the US: A life course health development approach." *Social Science & Medicine* 74(5): 671-73.

Hammond, W. P., D. Matthews, D. Mohottige, A. Agyemang and G. Corbie-Smith. 2010. "Masculinity, medical mistrust, and preventive health services delays among community-dwelling African-American men." *Journal of General Internal Medicine* 25(12): 1300-8.

Haney, Lynne and Miranda March. 2003. "Married fathers and caring daddies: Welfare reform and the discursive politics of paternity." *Social Problems* 50(4): 461-81.

Hayward, Mark D., Toni P. Miles, Eileen M. Crimmins and Yu Yang. 2000. "The significance of socioeconomic status in explaining the racial gap in chronic health conditions." *American Sociological Review* 65(6): 910-30.

Henretta, John C. 2007. "Early childbearing, marital status, and women's health and mortality." *Journal of Health and Social Behavior* 48 (September): 254-66.

Hereford, Sonnie Wellington. 2011. *Beside the troubled waters: A black doctor remembers life, medicine, and civil rights in an Alabama town*. Tuscaloosa, AL: University of Alabama Press.

Hill, Shirley A. 1994. *Managing sickle-cell disease in low-income families*. Philadelphia. PA: Temple University Press.

Hill, Shirley A. 2005. *Black intimacies: A gender perspective on families and relationships*. Walnut Creek, CA: AltaMira Press.

Hill, Shirley A. 2006. "Marriage among African Americans: A gender perspective." *Journal of Comparative Family Studies* XXXVII(3): 421-40.

Hill, Shirley A. 2008. "African American mothers: Victimized, vilified, and valorized." In A. O'Reilly (ed) *Feminist mMothering* (pp 107-23). New York: SUNY.

Hill, Shirley A. 2009. "Cultural images and the health of African American women." *Gender & Society* 23(6): 733-46.

Hill, Shirley A., Mary K. Zimmerman and Michael Fox. 2002. "Rational choice in Medicaid managed care: A critique." *Journal of Poverty* 6(2): 37-59.

Hill, Terrence D., Catherine E. Ross and Ronald J. Angel. 2005. "Neighborhood disorder, psychophysiological distress, and health." *Journal of Health and Social Behavior* 46(2): 170-86.

Hine, Darlene Clark and Kathleen Thompson. 1998. *A shining thread of hope*. New York: Broadway Books.

Holloway, Pippa. 2014. *Living in infamy: Felon disfranchisement and the history of American citizenship*. New York and Oxford: Oxford University Press.

Holt, Cheryl L. and Stephanie M. McClure. 2006. "Perceptions of religion-health connection among African American church members." *Qualitative Health Research* 16(2): 268-81.

House, James S. 2001. "Understanding social factors and inequalities in health: 20th century progress and 21st century prospects." *Journal of Health and Social Behavior* 43(2): 125-42.

Humphreys, Margaret. 2008. *Intensely human: The health of the black soldier in the American Civil War*. Baltimore, MD: Johns Hopkins University Press.

Hutchinson, Janis Faye. 1999. "The Hip Hop generation: African American male-female relationships in a nightclub setting." *Journal of Black Studies* 30(1): 62-84.

Illich, Ivan. 1976. *Medical nemesis*. New York: Random House.

Jackson, Grace L., David Kennedy, Thomas N. Bradbury and Benjamin R. Karney. 2014. "A social network comparison of low-income Black and White newlywed couples." *Journal of Marriage and Family* 76 (October): 967-82.

Jackson, Jerrold M., Puja Seth, Ralph J. DiClemente and Anne Lin. 2015. "Association of depressive symptoms and substance use with risky sexual behavior and sexually transmitted infections among African American female adolescents seeking sexual health care." *American Journal of Public Health* 105(10): 2137-42.

Jenkins, Candice M. 2007. *Private lives, proper relations*. Minneapolis, MN: University of Minnesota Press.

John, Daphne and Beth Anne Shelton. 1997. "The production of gender among Black and White women and men: The case of household labor." *Sex Roles* 36(3/4): 171-93.

Johnson, Patrik. 2016. "In poor neighborhoods, is it better to fix up or move out?" *Christian Science Monitor*, April 4.

Jones, Charisse and Kumea Shorter-Gooden. 2003. *Shifting: The double lives of black women in America*. New York: HarperCollins.

Jones, Jacqueline. 1985. *Labor of love, labor of sorrow: Black women, work, and the family from slavery to the present*. New York: Basic Books.

Jones, Nikki. 2010. *Between good and ghetto: African American girls and inner-city violence*. New Brunswick, NJ: Rutgers University Press.

Journal of the American Medical Association. 1906. "The negro brain." XLVII(20): 1660.

Klonoff, Elizabeth A. and Hope Landrine. 2000. "Is skin color a marker for racial discrimination? Explaining the skin color–hypertension relationship." *Journal of Behavioral Medicine* 23(4): 329-38.

Koball, Heather. 1998. "Have African American men become less committed to marriage? Explaining the twentieth century racial cross-over in men's marriage timing." *Demography* 35(2): 251-58.

Kogan, Steven M., Tianyi Yu and Geoffrey L. Brown. 2016. "Romantic relationship commitment behavior among emerging adult African American men." *Journal of Marriage and Family*. doi: 10.1111/jomf.12293

Kohn, Melvin L. 1963. "Social-class and parent-child relationships." *American Journal of Sociology* 63: 471-80.

Koos, Earl. 1954. *The health of Regionville*. New York: Columbia University Press.

Kornrich, Sabino. 2009. "Entrepreneurship as economic detour? Client segregation by race and class and the Black–White earnings gap among physicians." *Work and Occupations* 36(4): 400-31.

Kwate, Naa Oyo A. and Ilan H. Meyer. 2010. "The myth of meritocracy and African American health." *American Journal of Public Health* 100(10): 1831-4.

Ladner, Joyce A. and Ruby M. Gourdine. 1984. "Intergenerational teenage motherhood: Some preliminary findings" *Sage: A Scholarly Journal on Black Women* 1: 22-4.

Landry, Bart. 2000. *Black working wives: Pioneers of the American family revolution*. Berkeley, CA: University of California Press.

LaPierre, Tracey A. and Shirley A. Hill. 2013. "Examining status discrepant marriages and marital quality at the intersections of gender, race, and class." *Advances in Gender Research* 17(1): 115-38.

Lareau, Annette. 2003. *Unequal childhoods: Class, race, and family life.* Berkeley, CA: University of California Press.

Lee, Hedwig, Kathleen Mullan Harris and Penny Gordon-Larsen. 2009. "Life course perspective on the links between poverty and obesity during the transition to young adulthood." *Population Research and Policy Review* 28(4): 505-32.

Leininger, Lindsey and Helen Levy. 2015. "Child health and access to medical care." *The Future of Children* 25(1): 65-90.

Letiecq, Bethany L., Sandra J. Bailey and Fonda Porterfield. 2008. "'We have no rights, we get no help': The legal and policy dilemmas facing grandparent caregivers." *Journal of Family Issues* 29(8): 995-1012.

Levin, Jeff. 2009. "How faith heals: A theoretical model." *Explore* 5(2): 77-96.

Lim, Sungwoo and Tiffany Harris. 2015. "Neighborhood contributions to racial and ethnic disparities in obesity among New York City adults." *American Journal of Public Health* 105(1): 159-65.

Lincoln, Karen D., Linda M. Chatters and Robert Joseph Taylor. 2005. "Social support, traumatic events, and depressive symptoms among African Americans." *Journal of Marriage and Family* 67 (August): 754-66.

Link, Bruce G. and Jo Phelan. 1995. "Social conditions as fundamental causes of disease." *Journal of Health and Social Behavior* Extra Issue: 80-94.

Logan, Enid. 1999. "The wrong race, committing crime, doing drugs, and maladjusted for motherhood: The nation's fury over 'crack babies'." *Social Justice* 26(1): 115-38.

Long, Gretchen. 2012. *Doctoring freedom: The politics of African American medical care in slavery and emancipation.* Chapel Hill, NC: University of North Carolina Press.

Lukachko, Alicia, Mark L. Hatzenbuehler and Katherine M. Keyes. 2014. "Structural racism and myocardial infarction in the United States." *Social Science & Medicine* 103: 42-50.

Lumpkins, Crystal Y., K. Allen Greiner, Christine Daley, Natabhona M. Mabachi and Kris Neuhaus. 2014. "Promoting health behavior from the pulpit: Clergy share their perspectives on effective health communication in the African American church." *Journal of Religion and Health* 52: 1093-107.

Lutfey, Karen and Jeremy Freese. 2005. "Toward some fundamentals of fundamental causality: Socioeconomic status and health in the routine clinic visit for diabetes." *American Journal of Sociology* 110(5): 1326-72.

Mackler, Jennifer S., Rachael T. Kelleher, Lilly Shanahan, Susan D. Calkins, Susan P. Keane and Marion O'Brien. 2015. "Parenting stress, parental reactions, and externalizing behavior from ages 4 to 10." *Journal of Marriage and Family* 77(2): 388-406.

Majors, Richard and Janet Macini Billson. 1992. *Cool pose: The dilemmas of black manhood in America.* New York: Lexington Books.

Mandara, Jelani, Jamie S. Johnston, Carolyn B. Murray and Fatima Varner. 2008. "Marriage, money, and African American mothers' self-esteem." *Journal of Marriage and Family* 70 (December): 1188-99.

Marmot, Michael. 2015. *The health gap: The challenge of an unequal world.* New York: Bloomsbury.

Martin, Stephen A., Kenn Harris and Brian W. Jack. 2015. "The health of young African American men." *Journal of the American Medical Association* 313(14): 1415-16.

Maselko, Joanna, Cayce Hughes and Rose Cheney. 2011. "Religious social capital: Its measurement and utility in the study of the social determinants of health." *Social Science & Medicine* 73: 759-67.

Massoglia, Michael. 2008a. "Incarceration, health, and racial disparities in health." *Law & Society Review* 42(2): 275-306.

Massoglia, Michael. 2008b. "Incarceration as exposure: The prison, infectious disease, and other stress-related illnesses." *Journal of Health and Social Behavior* 49(1): 56-71.

Masters, Ryan K., Bruce G. Link and Jo C. Phelan. 2015. "Trends in education gradient of 'preventable' mortality: A test of fundamental cause theory." *Social Science & Medicine* 127.

McClintock, Elizabeth Aura. 2010. "When does race matter? Race, sex, and dating at an elite university." *Journal of Marriage and Family* 72(1): 45-72.

McCormack, Karen. 2005. "Stratified reproduction and poor women's resistance." *Gender & Society* 19(5): 660-79.

McLanahan, Sara and Christine Percheski. 2008. "Family structure and the reproduction of inequalities." *Annual Review of Sociology* 34: 257-76.

McLanahan, Sara and Dona Schwartz. 2002. "Life without father: What happens to the children." *Contexts* 1(1): 35-41.

McLoyd, V. C., A. M. Cauce, D. Takeuchi and L. Wilson. 2000. "Marital processes and parental socialization in families of color: A decade review." *Journal of Marriage and the Family* 62(4): 1070-93.

McQuillan, Julia, Arthur L. Greil, Karina M. Shreffler and Andrew V. Bedrous. 2015. "The importance of motherhood and fertility intentions among US women." *Sociological Perspectives* 58(1): 20-35.

Mechanic, David. 1995. "Sociological dimensions of illness behavior." *Social Science & Medicine* 41: 1207-16.

Mechanic, David and Donna A. McAlpine. 2010. "Sociology of health care reform: Building on research and analysis to improve health care." *Journal of Health and Social Behavior* 51(S)(1): S147-S59.

Mickelson, Kristin D. and Jessica L. Demmings. 2009. "The impact of support network substitution on low-income women's health: Are minor children beneficial substitutes?" *Social Science & Medicine* 68: 80-8.

Milardo, R. M. and A. Graham. 2000. "Social networks and marital relationships." In R. M. Milardo and S. Duck (eds) *Families as relationships* (Chapter 3). New York: John Wiley & Sons.

Miller, Richard B., Cody S. Hollist, Joseph Olsen and David Law. 2013. "Marital quality and health over 20 years: A growth curve analysis." *Journal of Marriage and Family* 75(3): 667-80.

Mitchell, Stephanie J., Amy Lewin, Ivor B. Horn, Dawn Valentine, Kathy Sanders-Phillips and Jill G. Joseph. 2010. "How does violence exposure affect the psychological health and parenting of young African-American mothers?" *Social Science & Medicine* 70(4): 526-33.

Mollborn, Stefanie, Laurie James-Hawkins, Elizabeth Lawrence and Paula Fomby. 2014. "Health lifestyles in early childhood." *Journal of Health and Social Behavior* 55(4): 386-402.

Morais, Herbert M. 1968. *The history of the Negro in medicine.* New York: Publishers Company, Inc.

Morgen, Sandra. 2002. *Into our own hands: The Women's Health Movement in the United States, 1969-1990.* New Brunswick, NJ: Rutgers University Press.

Morris, Martina, Ann E. Kurth, Deven T. Hamilton, James Moody and Steve Wakefield. 2009. "Concurrent partnerships and HIV prevalence disparities by race: Linking science and public health practice." *American Journal of Public Health* 99(6): 1023-33.

Moynihan, Daniel Patrick. 1965. *The Negro family: The case for national action.* Washington, DC: Office of Policy Planning and Research.

Muennig, Peter and Michael Murphy. 2011. "Does racism affect health?" *Journal of Health Politics, Policy and Law* 36(1): 187-214.

Muller, Christopher. 2012. "Northward migration and the rise of racial disparity in American incarceration, 1880-1950." *American Journal of Sociology* 118(2): 281-326.

Murphy, Sean. 2016. "Police officer who raped gets 263 years in prison." *New York Times* 2A.

Murray, C. 1984. *Losing ground: American social policy 1950-1980*. New York: Basic Books.

Musick, Marc A., James S. House and David R. Williams. 2004. "Attendance at religious services and mortality in a national sample." *Journal of Health and Social Behavior* 45(2): 198-213.

Nomaguchi, Kei and Amanda N. House. 2013. "Racial-ethnic disparities in maternal parenting stress: The role of structural disadvantage and parenting values." *Journal of Health and Social Behavior* 54(3): 386-404.

Okie, Susan. 2009. "The epidemic that wasn't." *The New York Times* 158: D1(L).

Oliver, Melvin L. and Thomas M. Shapiro. 1995. *Black wealth/White wealth: A new perspective on racial inequality*. New York: Routledge.

Oliver, Melvin and Thomas M. Shapiro. 2001. "Wealth and racial stratification." In N. J. Smelser, W. J. Wilson and F. Mitchell (eds) *America becoming: Racial trends and their consequences* (pp 222-51). Washington, DC: National Academy Press.

Oliver, Melvin L. and Thomas M. Shapiro. 2008. "Sub-prime as a Black catastrophe." *The American Prospect*, October, A9-A11.

Oppenheimer, Gerald M. 2001. "Paradigm lost: Race, ethnicity, and search for a new population taxonomy." *American Journal of Public Health* 91(7): 1049-55.

Osborne, Cynthia and Sara McLanahan. 2007. "Partnership instability and child well-being." *Journal of Marriage and Family* 69 (November): 1065-83.

Outley, Corliss Wilson. 2006. "A content analysis of health and physical activity messages marketed to African American children during after-school television programming." *Archives of Pediatric and Adolescent Medicine* 150 (April): 432-35.

Owens, Leslie Howard. 1976. *This species of property: Slave life and culture in the Old South*. New York: Oxford University Press.

Pampel, Fred C., Patrick M. Krueger and Justin T. Denney. 2010. "Socioeconomic disparities in health behaviors." *Annual Review of Sociology* 36: 349-70.

Paquette, Danielle. 2015. "The sex lives of rich and poor women are remarkably similar – until it comes to birth control." *Washington Post* March 15.

Parker-Pope, Tara. 2010. "Is marriage good for your health?" *New York Times*.

Pattillo-McCoy, Mary. 1999. *Black picket fences: Privilege and peril among the black middle class.* Chicago, IL and London: University of Chicago Press.

Pavalko, Eliza K. and Jennifer Caputo. 2013. "Social inequality and health across the life course." *American Behavioral Scientist* 57(8): 1040-56.

Pazol, K., A. A. Creanga, K. D. Burley and D. Jamieson. 2014 "Abortion surveillance US 2011." Vol 63. Atlanta, GA: Center for Disease Control and Prevention.

Pearlin, Leonard I. 1989. "The sociological study of stress." *Journal for Marriage and Family* 30: 241-56.

Pearlin, Leonard I., Elizabeth G. Menaghan, Morton A. Lieberman and Joseph T. Mullan. 1981. "The stress process." *Journal of Health and Social Behavior* 22(4): 337-56.

Peek, Monica E., Judith V. Sayad and Ronald Markwardt. 2008. "Fear, fatalism and breast cancer screening in low-income African-American women: The role of clinicians and the health care system." *Journal of General Internal Medicine* 23(11): 1847-53.

Perry, Armon Rashard. 2013. "African American men's attitudes toward marriage." *Journal of Black Studies* 44(2): 182-202.

Pescosolido, Bernice A. 1992. "Beyond rational choice: The social dynamics of how people seek help." *American Journal of Sociology* 97: 1096-138.

Pflieger, Jacqueline C., Emily Cook, Linda Niccolai and Christian Connell. 2013. "Racial/ethnic differences in patterns of sexual risk behavior and rates of sexually transmitted infections among female young adults." *American Journal of Public Health* 103(5): 903-09.

Phelan, Jo, Bruce G. Link and Parisa Tehranifar. 2010. "Social conditions as fundamental causes of health inequalities: Theory, evidence, and policy implications." *Journal of Health and Social Behavior* 51: S28-S40.

Pickett, Kate E. and Richard G. Wilkinson. 2015. "Income inequality and health: A causal review." *Social Science & Medicine* 128 (March): 316-26.

Plescia, Marcus, Harry Herrick and LaTonya Chavis. 2008. "Improving health behaviors in an African American community: The Charlotte Racial and Ethnic Approaches to Community Health Project." *American Journal of Public Health* 98(9): 1678-84.

Powell, T. O. 1896. "The increase of insanity and tuberculois in the southern Negro since 1860, and its alliance, and some supposed causes." *Journal of the American Medical Association* XXVII(23): 1185-6.

Quadagno, Jill. 2000. "Promoting civil rights through the welfare state: How Medicare integrated southern hospitals." *Social Problems* 47(1): 68-89.

Quadagno, Jill. 2009. "Why the United States has no national health insurance: Stakeholder mobilization against the welfare state, 1945-1996." In P. Conrad (ed) *The sociology of health and illness: Critical perspectives* (pp 301-20). New York: Worth.

Quadagno, Jill. 2010. "Institutions, interest groups, and ideology: An agenda for the sociology of health care reform." *Journal of Health and Social Behavior* 51(2): 125-36.

Ravenell, Joseph E., Eric E. Whitaker and Waldo Johnson. 2008. "According to him: Barriers to healthcare about African-American men." *Journal of the National Medical Association* 100(10): 1153-60.

Roberts, Dorothy. 1997. *Killing the black body: Race, reproduction, and the meaning of liberty.* New York: Pantheon Books.

Robinson, Russell K. 2009. "Racing the closet." *Stanford Law Review* 61(6): 1463-533.

Roebuck, Julian and Robert Quan. 1976. "Health care practices in the American Deep South." In R. Wallis and P. Morely (eds) *Marginal medicine.* New York: The Free Press.

Romero, Edna, Maryse H. Richards, Patrick Harrison, James Garbarino and Michaela Mozley. 2015. "The role of neighborhood in the development of aggression in urban African American youth: A multilevel analysis." *American Journal of Community Psychology* 56: 156-69.

Roschelle, Anne R. 1997. *No more kin: Exploring race, class, and gender in family networks.* Thousand Oaks, CA: Sage.

Rosenstock, Irwin. 1966. "Why people use health services." *The Milbank Memorial Fund Quarterly* 44(3): 94-127.

Rosenthal, Lisa and Marci Lobel. 2011. "Explaining racial disparities in adverse birth outcomes: Unique sources of stress for Black American women." *Social Science & Medicine* 72: 977-83.

Rosmarin, David H., Joseph S. Bigda-Peyton, Sarah J. Kertz and Nasya Smith. 2013. "A test of faith in God and treatment: The relationship of belief in God to psychiatric treatment outcomes." *Journal of Affective Disorders* 146: 441-46.

Ross, Catherine E. 2000. "Neighborhood disadvantage and adult depression." *Journal of Health and Social Behavior* 41(2): 177-87.

Ross, Catherine E. and John Mirowsky. 2009. "Neighborhood disorder, subjective alienation, and distress." *Journal of Health and Social Behavior* 50(1): 49-64.

Rossin-Slater, Maya. 2015. "Promoting health in early childhood." *The Future of Children* 25(1): 35-64.

Rowland, Michael L. and E. Paulette Isaac-Savage. 2014. "As I see it: A study of African American pastors' views on health and health education in the Black church." *Journal of Religious Health* 53: 1091-101.

Rugh, Jacob S., Len Albright and Douglas S. Massey. 2015. "Race, space, and cumulative disadvantage: A case study of the subprime lending collapse." *Social Problems* 62(2): 186–218.

Sarkisian, Natalia and Kathleen Gerson. 2004. "Kin support among Blacks and Whites: Race and family organization." *American Sociological Review* 69 (December): 812-37.

Savitt, Todd L. 1978. *Medicine and slavery: The diseases and health care of Blacks in Antebellum Virginia.* Chicago, IL: University of Illinois Press.

Savitt, Todd L. 2005. "Black health on the plantation: Owners, the enslaved, and physicians." *OAH Magazine of History* 19(5): 14-16.

Schmeer, Kammi K. 2012. "Family structure and obesity in early childhood." *Social Science Research* 41: 820-32.

Schnittker, Jason and Andrea John. 2007. "Enduring stigma: The long-term effects of incarceration on health." *Journal of Health and Social Behavior* 48(2): 115-30.

Schnittker, Jason, Michael Massoglia and Christopher Uggen. 2012. "Out and down: Incarceration and psychiatric disorders." *Journal of Health and Social Behavior* 53(4): 448-64.

Schulz, Amy J. and Lora Bex Lempert. 2004. "Being part of the world: Detroit women's perceptions of health and the social environment." *Journal of Contemporary Ethnography* 33(4): 437-65.

Schulz, Amy, David Williams, Barbara Israel, Adam Becker, Edith Parker, Sherman A. James and James Jackson. 2000. "Unfair treatment, neighborhood effects, and mental health in the Detroit metropolitan area." *Journal of Health and Social Behavior* 41(3): 314-32.

Seccombe, Karen. 2007. *Families in poverty,* New York: Pearson Education.

Sellers, Sherrill L. and Harold W. Neighbors. 2008. "Effects of goal-striving stress on the mental health of Black Americans." *Journal of Health and Social Behavior* 49(1): 92-103.

Sewell, Abigail, Kevin A. Jefferson and Hedwig Lee. 2016. "Living under surveillance: Gender, psychological distress, and stop-question-and frisk policing in New York City." *Social Science & Medicine* 159: 1-13.

Shariff-Marco, Salma, Ann C. Klassen and Janice V. Bowie. 2010. "Racial/ethnic differences in self-reported racism and its association with cancer-related health behaviors." *American Journal of Public Health* 100(2): 364-74.

Shea, Steven and Mindy Thompson Fullilove. 1985. "Entry of Black and other minority students to US medical schools." *New England Journal of Medicine* 313(3): 933-40.

Shim, Janet K. 2010. "Cultural health capital: A theoretical approach to understanding health care interactions and the dynamics of unequal treatment." *Journal of Health and Social Behavior* 51(1): 1-15.

Shryock, Richard Harrison. 1966. *Medicine in America: Historical essays.* Baltimore, MD: Johns Hopkins University Press.

Siefert, Kristine, Colleen M. Heflin, Mary E. Corcoran and David R. Williams. 2004. "Food insufficiency and physical and mental health in a longitudinal survey of welfare recipients." *Journal of Health and Social Behavior* 45(2): 171-86.

Skloot, Rebecca. 2010. *The immortal life of Henrietta Lacks.* London: Macmillan.

Smedley, Brian D. and Adrienne Y. Stith. 2003. *Unequal treatment: Confronting racial and ethnic disparities in health care.* Washington, DC: National Academies Press.

Smith, Susan L. 1995. *Sick and tired of being sick and tired: Black women's health activism in America, 1890-1950.* Philadelphia, PA: University of Pennsylvania Press.

Smith, D. B. 1999. *Health care divided: Race and healing a nation.* Ann Arbor, MI: University of Michigan Press.

Solinger, Rickie. 2005. *Pregnancy and power: A short history of reproductive politics in America.* New York: New York University Press.

Spence, Naomi J., Daniel E. Adkins and Matthew E. Dupre. 2011. "Racial differences in depression trajectories among older women: Socioeconomic, family, and health influences." *Journal of Health and Social Behavior* 52(4): 444-59.

Stampp, Kenneth M. 1956. *The peculiar institution: Slavery in the Antebellum South.* New York: Vintage Books.

Stanik, Christine E. and Chalandra M. Bryant. 2012. "Marital quality of newlywed African American couples: Implications for egalitarian gender role dynamics." *Sex Roles* 66: 256-67.

Stanik, Christine E., Susan M. McHale and Ann C. Crouter. 2013. "Gender dynamics predict changes in marital love among African American couples." *Journal of Marriage and Family* 75(4): 795-807.

Staples, Robert. 2006. *Exploring Black sexuality.* Lanham, MD: Rowman & Littlefield.

Starr, Paul. 1982. *The social transformation of American medicine*. New York: Basic Books.

Starr, Paul. 2011. *Remedy and reaction: The peculiar American struggle over health care reform*. New Haven, CT and London, UK: Yale University Press.

Stepanikova, Irena, Stefanie Mollborn, Karen S. Cook, David H. Thom and Roderick M. Kramer. 2006. "Patients' race, ethnicity, language, and trust in a physician." *Journal of Health and Social Behavior* 47(4): 390-405.

Stone, Deborah. 2005. "How market ideology guarantees racial inequality." In J. A. Morone and L. R. Jacobs (eds) *Healthy, wealthy, and fair: Health care and the good society* (pp 65-91). New York and Oxford, UK: Oxford University Press.

Strauss, Robert. 1957. "The nature and status of medical sociology." *American Sociological Review* 22(1): 200-04.

Stueve, Ann, Lydia O'Donnell and Bruce Link. 2001. "Gender differences in risk factors for violent behavior among economically disadvantaged African American and Hispanic young adolescents." *International Journal of Law and Psychiatry* 24(4-5): 539-57.

Suchman, Edward A. 1965. "Social patterns of illness and medical care." *Journal of Health and Social Behavior* 6: 2-16.

Sugarmann, Josh. 2014. "Murder rate for black Americans is four times the national average." *Huffington Post* January 31.

Summers, Martin. 2014. "Diagnosing the ailments of Black citizenship: African American physicians and the politics of mental illness, 1895-1940." In L. B. Green, J. McKiernan-Gonzalez and M. Summers (eds) *Precarious prescriptions: Contested histories of race and health in North America* (pp 91-114). Minneapolis, MN: University of Minnesota Press.

Swidler, Ann. 1986. "Culture in action: Symbols and strategies." *American Sociological Review* 51 (April): 273-86.

Szasz, Thomas. 1961. *The myth of mental illness: Foundations of a theory of personal conduct*. New York: Hoeber-Harper.

Tavernise, Sabrina. 2015. "Rise in suicide by black children surprises." *New York Times*, May 18.

Thomas, Karen Kruse. 2011. *Deluxe Jim Crow: Civil rights and American health policy, 1935-1954*. Athens, GA: University of Georgia Press.

Thomson, Elizabeth, Thomas L. Hanson and S. McLanahan. 1994. "Family structure and child well-being: Economic resources vs parental behaviors." *Social Forces* 73(1): 221-42.

Trenholm, Christopher, Barbara Devaney, Kenneth Fortson, Melissa Clark, Lisa Quay Bridgespan and Justin Wheeler. 2008. "Impacts of abstinence education on teen sexual activity, risk of pregnancy, and risk of sexually transmitted diseases." *Journal of Policy Analysis and Management* 27(2): 255-76.

Uggen, Christopher, Jeff Manza and Melissa Thompson. 2006. "Citizenship, democracy, and the civic reintegration of criminal offenders." *Annals of the American Academy of Political and Social Science* 605: 281-310.

Umberson, Debra, Hui Liu and Daniel Powers. 2009. "Marital status, marital transitions, and body weight." *Journal of Health and Social Behavior* 50 (September): 327-43.

Umberson, Debra, Kristi Williams, Patricia A. Thomas, Hui Liu and Mieke Beth Thomeer. 2014. "Race, gender, and chains of disadvantage: Childhood adversity, social relationships, and health." *Journal of Health and Social Behavior* 55(1): 20-8.

van Cleue, Nicole Gonzalez. 2016. "Chicago's racist cops and racist courts." *New York Times*, April 14.

van Ryan, Michelle and Jane Burke. 2000. "The effect of patient race and socio-economic status on physicians' perceptions of patients." *Social Science & Medicine* 50: 813-28.

Vartanian, Thomas P. and Linda Houser. 2010. "The effects of childhood neighborhood conditions on self-reports of adult health." *Journal of Health and Social Behavior* 51(3): 291-306.

Villatoro, Alice P. and Carol S. Aneshensel. 2014. "Family influences on the use of mental health services among African Americans." *Journal of Health and Social Behavior* 55(2): 161-80.

Waitzkin, H. 1983. *The second sickness: Contradictions of capitalist health care*. New York: Free Press.

Wakefield, Sara and Christopher Wildeman. 2014. *Children of the prison boom: Mass incarceration and the future of American inequality*. Oxford/ New York: Oxford University Press.

Walker, Alice. 1970. *The third life of Grange Copeland*. Orlando, FL: Harcourt, Inc.

Walker, Renee E. and Melanie Gordon. 2013. "The use of lifestyle and behavioral modification approaches in obesity interventions for Black women: A literature review." *Health Education & Behavior* XX(X): 1-17.

Walton, Emily. 2009. "Residential segregation and birth weight among racial and ethnic minorities in the United States." *Journal of Health and Social Behavior* 50 (December): 427-42.

Ward, Earlist C., Le Ondra Clark and A Heidrich. 2009. "African American women's beliefs, coping behaviors, and barriers to seeking mental health services." *Qualitative Health Research* 19(11): 1589-601.

Warren, John Robert, Laurie Knies, Steven Haas and Elaine M. Hernandez. 2012. "The impact of childhood sickness on adult socioeconomic outcomes: Evidence from late 19th century America." *Social Science & Medicine* 75(8): 1531-38.

Watson, Wilbur H. 1999. *Against the odds: Blacks in the profession of medicine in the US.* New Brunswick, NJ: Transaction.

Weitz, Rose. 2013. *The sociology of health, illness, and health care: A critical approach.* Boston, MA: Wadsworth.

Western, Bruce and Katherine Beckett. 1999. "How unregulated is the US labor market? The penal system as a labor market institution." *American Journal of Sociology* 104(4): 1030-60.

Western, Bruce, Anthony A. Braga, Jaclyn Davis and Catherine Sirois. 2015. "Stress and hardship after prison." *American Journal of Sociology* 120(5): 1512-47.

Wildeman, Christopher and Bruce Western. 2010. "Incarceration in fragile families." *The Future of Children* 20(2): 157-77.

Wildeman, C., J. Schnittker and K. Turney. 2012. "Despair by association? The mental health of mothers with children by recently incarcerated fathers." *American Sociological Review* 77(2): 216-43.

Williams, David R. 2012. "Miles to go before we sleep: Racial inequities in health." *Journal of Health and Social Behavior* 53(3): 279-95.

Williams, David R. and Selina A. Mohammed. 2013. "Racism and health 1. Pathways and scientific evidence." *American Behavioral Scientist* 57(8): 1152-73.

Williams, David R. and Michelle Sternthal. 2010. "Understanding racial-ethnic disparities in health: Sociological contributions." *Journal of Health and Social Behavior* 51: S15-S27.

Wilson, William J. 1978. *The declining significance of race: Blacks and changing American institutions.* Chicago, IL: University of Chicago Press.

Wysong, Earl, Robert Perrucci and David Wright. 2014. *The new class society: Goodbye American dream?* Lanham, MD: Rowman & Littlefield.

Xanthos, Clare, Henrie M. Treadwell and Kisha B. Holden. 2012. "Introduction to social determinants of health among African-American men." In H. M. Treadwell, C. Xanthos and K. B. Holden (eds) *Social determinants of health among African-American men* (pp 1-21). San Francisco, CA: Jossey-Bass.

Young, Alford. 2004. *The lives of marginalized Black men: Making sense of mobility, opportunity, and future life chances*. Princeton, NJ: Princeton University Press.

Zborowski, Mark. 1952. "Cultural components in responses to pain." *Journal of Social Issues* 8: 16-30.

Zimmerman, Mary K. and Shirley A. Hill. 2000. "Re-forming gendered health care: An assessment of change." *International Journal of Health Services* 30(4): 769-93.

Zola, Irving Kenneth. 1966. "Culture and symptoms – an analysis of a patient's presenting complaints." *American Sociological Review* 31(5): 615-30.

Index